Lose Weight
Peacefully

Discover your ideal weight eating food you love

Jen Gallagher

ESSENTIAL OIL GODDESS

First published in Australia by Essential Oil Goddess in 2009
www.essential-oil-goddess.com
www.loseweightpeacefully.com

copyright © Janette Gallagher, 2009

Project Management Best Legenz www.bestlegenz.com.au

National Library of Australia Cataloguing-in-Publication entry

Author:	Gallagher, Jen
Title:	Lose weight peacefully / Jen Gallagher.
ISBN:	9780980711707 (pbk.)
Subjects:	Weight loss.
	Weight loss--Psychological aspects.
	Self-realization.

Dewey Number: 613.25

Distribution in Australia and New Zealand: Dennis Jones & Associates, Unit 1, 10 Melrich Road, Bayswater, Victoria 3153; www.dennisjones.com.au +61 (0)3 9762 9100

Editor: Ian Demack
Cover design: Best Legenz www.bestlegenz.com.au
Internal design: Best Legenz www.bestlegenz.com.au
Printed in Australia by McPherson's Printing Group

To world peace.
It begins with self-reflection.

Contents

Acknowledgments

I walked into the first Women's Publishing Network Non Fiction Writers' Group meeting on 13 March 2009, not ever knowing that I would have written and published my book by the end of 2009. It was that day that I met my mentor—the wonderful Jane Teresa Anderson. Without you Jane this book would never have become a reality. My heartfelt thanks goes out to you.

To the lovely Bev Ryan and all the inspirational women at the Non Fiction Writers' Group in Brisbane: thank you for sharing your wisdom, hopes and dreams as I have shared with you.

To Helen Elward and Bernice Kesbah of Best Legenz: thank you for your patience, dedication and meticulous approach to self-publishing that has given me this awesome book.

To Ian Demack—editor extraordinaire—your objectivity and attention to detail is perfect. Thank you so much.

To my beautiful partner Wai, thank you for listening to my ups and downs and being there to support me every step of the way.

To my two children, I love you and thank you for being there and being you.

To my wonderful friend Pam, thank you from the bottom of my heart, for taking the time to offer valuable suggestions, to make my book the best it can be. Your friendship and support are a blessing to me.

To my fantastic friends Caro and Karen for the feedback and encouragement to keep going.

To Tina-Renae for the stunning artwork for Essential Oil Goddess.

To all my past and present clients: thank you for giving me the inspiration to write *Insights into Peace*.

To the contributors to this book, thank you for being part of my journey.

And to you—thank you for joining me on this journey. I wish you peace, love and happiness.

Introduction

"Who wants to lose weight?" I was at a conference recently where the speaker was discussing nutrition. There were six hundred people in the audience, and when he asked this question about five hundred and ninety hands went up. I glanced around the audience and noticed there were people of all sizes. I thought to myself, "Why have so many people got their hands up?" Most of the five hundred and ninety people were not overweight. In fact, these people had gathered for a natural health conference and many were dedicated practitioners. My quick scan of the room told me that most people believe they need to lose weight, regardless of their size.

The question of losing weight got me thinking. I asked my size 10 girlfriend, "Do you want to lose weight?" She astounded me with her answer, "Well, yes, a little" she replied. I questioned her further. "Because I would feel more comfortable a few kilos lighter, more energetic, and feel better about myself," she explained. Then she said, "I would feel more in control." I asked her, "In control of what?" She replied, "When I am out of control I put energy into everyone except myself." So I wanted to know how her life would be different if she lost weight. After some thought, she replied "It wouldn't."

My friend believed that she could achieve some control in her life by dieting. Unless she aimed for perfection, she felt out of control. She believed that she would feel better if she lost weight. It didn't occur to her that she should address her need to put other people ahead of herself. By focussing on food and dieting, she was ignoring the real question. What was really eating her?

So why do so many people want to lose weight? They may want to look good, feel good or be healthy. But this doesn't explain why we are obsessed with food and dieting. Every day, we are bombarded with images of so-called perfection in the media and advertising, represented by skinny models and celebrities. We believe this is something to attain. When our lives are better—when we have lost the weight—then we too can attain perfection. It is an impossible goal. While trying to achieve it we miss out on all the other aspects of life. Our focus is so skewed we don't see the real picture.

The real picture is the life we have now, regardless of our weight. Once we focus on living, rather than on dieting and losing weight, we become happier and more confident. We lose weight easily. Food loses its power and we don't need to control it. We just need to understand ourselves and our feelings. By acknowledging our feelings, we learn compassion. We replace self-criticism with self-awareness. We open our hearts to the feeling of peace. Peacefulness can lead us to a new life where food and dieting are not the centre of our attention. Instead, we focus on what we can do with our lives once we are freed from that old obsession with food. As a bonus, we lose weight gracefully, and attain our ideal weight.

We have often been told that we are an obese nation, and that we need to lose weight. At the same time, we are offered more food than we are capable of eating.

We are seduced by high fat, high sugar and high carbohydrate foods, with a liberal splash of chemicals and additives. Advertising tells us that these are delicious and delectable foods, and that we deserve to treat ourselves. On the one hand, we want to gorge ourselves with this food. On the other, we resist, believing that we are in control of our diets. In fact we are like a tightly wound spring. Every time we deny ourselves a treat, we wind the spring tighter and tighter, until finally we can't hold it down any longer and all hell breaks loose. Suddenly we find ourselves on a binge, telling ourselves how fat and greedy we are and blaming it all on the food and our weight. All along, though, we ignore the real question: what is really eating us?

We also use food as a substitute for feeling good or as a reward. Rewarding ourselves with treats reinforces the connection between food and our feelings. We offer food to others, suggesting they treat themselves just this once, because we know no other way to give. When there are things missing from our lives, food is everywhere, waiting to fill the void. And if food is not filling the void, we are obsessing about controlling our temptation.

What happens when food is no longer the obsession? We don't know how to fill the empty space within. Food can give us not only the physical feeling of fullness but a temporary feeling of spiritual fulfilment as well. Food numbs us so much that we don't have to think about the real issues in our lives. Instead, we worry about how much we ate and enter into a cycle of destructive self-criticism. We vow once again to diet and so the cycle continues.

We believe that losing weight will give us the magical answer to all our problems. Once we lose weight we can do the things we want to do and be who we want to be. Until we do lose the weight we don't allow our true desires and dreams to flourish. We put it off until we have lost the weight.

And then when our dreams don't eventuate we still have food, binging and our lack of will power during the diet to blame.

Many of us believe that losing weight is the real issue when it is really the struggle for perfection that stops us from performing at our best. As a result, we continue to compare ourselves with others, and hate ourselves for our imperfections. Only when we have lost the weight can we allow ourselves to do what we really want to do. The problem is that we rarely achieve that goal weight. And if by some miracle we do succeed, we find that food is still an issue—an obsession.

From a very young age I learnt that food was the one thing that I could rely on. I had been using it for all those years. My obsession with food and dieting was stopping me from living my life. My journey has taken me from the despair of food obsession to a feeling of peace with my life. A life where I do not need to use food as my crutch for living; a life where I don't need to rely on food to support me through pain, happiness or any emotion in between. My focus on food— whether dieting or binging—was always hiding my emotions underneath the layers of fat.

Imagine a life where you are at complete peace with the food you eat. You choose to eat when you are hungry and acknowledge your feelings instead of eating them. Your payoff is that you will return to your ideal weight and accept yourself for who you really are. Imagine spending no more time, energy and money on diets, on losing weight, or on your food obsession. In this book you will learn a new way to look at food as fuel for your body. You will learn to value yourself enough to put quality fuel into your body when you need it. You will also learn that food and feelings can be separated. You will finally set yourself free!

How to Use This Book

This book is divided into three sections. You can read the book from start to finish or choose the section that appeals to you. The first section is *My Story*. My story is not unique. It is the story of the pain of my childhood where I learned to use food to protect myself from perceived danger. It explains how I continued this pattern right through my teenage years to adulthood, when I began to sense who I really could be if I let go of food as my anchor. This sets the scene for my new thoughts on food, and how I came to realise that my food obsession had stopped me living my dreams and my life for so long.

The second section is *Diet to Peace*. It explains the transformation that took place when I finally realised that dieting and losing weight were not the answers to my problems. The second section gives specific examples of how to challenge your thinking when you feel that dieting is the only answer to your problems—it is not. The second section may be considered as a "how to live peacefully without food obsession and dieting" guide. Once you make the decision to change, the payoff is that you lose weight anyway because you are happy with who you are and don't need food to fill the void.

The third section contains the *Insights into Peace: Daily Practices*. This section allows you to "pick and choose" a practice that is right for you at any particular moment. For example, if you are craving a certain food, you may like to read Chapter 8—*Feelings*, and find an *Insight to Peace to* explore the emotions that are surfacing for you at that time. You may also choose to work through the practices in order to thoroughly explore how you connect food with your feelings and life. I suggest that you keep a journal specifically for working through these practices. You will experience growth while working on these practices, and your journal will help you to reflect on how far you have come.

The third section also includes the use of essential oils. I believe that essential oil scents can change your mood. Smell is the only sense where the receptor nerve endings are in direct contact with the outside world. Essential oil molecules are so small that they are able to bypass the blood-brain barrier and go directly to the brain via the sense of smell. Scientific research shows that essential oils are readily absorbed into the blood stream and that excellent absorption takes place through the nasal mucosa and lungs. Therefore, when inhaled, essential oils may stimulate the areas of the brain associated with memory and learning. They may also influence hormonal responses, and alter moods and feelings.

Each *Insight to Peace* contains a list of essential oils suitable for use during each practice. It is important that only therapeutic grade essential oils are used. Possible applications of the oils are explained in the *Appendix*. I believe that essential oils have been pivotal to the changes that have occurred in my life. I have finally ended my war with food, and found my peace. My background in aromatherapy has led me to explore the emotional applications of essential oils.

Essential oils have been connected with emotional applications for quite some time. I have trained in a form of emotional clearing using therapeutic grade essential oils. Our bodies have an astounding ability to relax and feel emotions. It is this work with the emotional applications of the oils that led me to include essential oils as part of the journey of self-discovery.

I also needed something tangible to work with when doing the *Insight into Peace* practices. For me essential oils provided me with a medium to access emotions and feelings, even when I felt blocked. Try them for yourself and see if they enhance your understanding of yourself. It did for me. Please see the *Resources* section for more information about accessing therapeutic grade essential oils.

This has been a personal journey for me to finally acknowledge that I was like the "living dead". I was not brave enough to live my life to the full. I have had my traumas in the past and have hidden behind food for many years, allowing it to become the main focus in my life. When I took away the food obsession I found so much more space to do what I want. We all have a life to be lived. I hope this book inspires you to give up dieting, honour yourself with food you love, and focus on the important things in life. As a consequence you will lose weight peacefully.

My Story

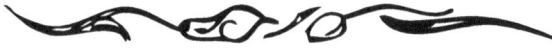

1

The Story So Far

WHO WOULD HAVE THOUGHT I would be writing a book about losing weight? I have struggled with my weight for as long as I can remember. I started my first diet when I was ten years old. The doctor told my mother that I needed to "lose some weight." The pictures tell the story. I didn't understand that my weight gain was due to eating too much or eating the wrong types of foods. I know now that I ate when I wasn't hungry. I was filling up on foods to feel better. Being full helped fill the emptiness inside.

I was constantly bullied, had an alcoholic father and never felt safe. I knew that something was not quite right, but I was too young to understand how I could feel so hurt by the people who loved me.

I was in pain at ten years old. I felt helpless and hopeless. The only way I could feel better was to eat until I was so full that I couldn't feel anything else. Food was my comfort and protection from the pain of the outside world. So I learnt from an early age that food was a quick, easy and accessible way to deal with pain. And because I didn't feel love from the people around me, I didn't love myself. I didn't know how to ask for help or speak up for myself when I was bullied or put down by my father.

Instead of finding a way to give me the love, help and support I needed, my mother took me to Weight Watchers. I guess this was the only way she knew how to express her love. I received two hugs from my mother in her lifetime that I remember. The first was when I was thirteen years old and got my first period. I was so shocked, I started crying and my mother hugged me. The second and last time was the day before she died. It was very hard for her to talk about emotions and she avoided it most of the time. She showed her love in other ways like providing me with food, especially when I didn't need it, when all I needed was a hug instead of layers of fat.

She was a good mum and wanted the best for me, making sure that I ate my allowance of liver each week and limiting my intake of hard cheese. Those were just a couple of the Weight Watchers rules in those days. I vividly remember the first week of that diet. My neighbour was having his tenth birthday party. He had a barbeque. I remember looking at the food and wanting—just wanting and feeling completely left out. I had to restrain myself. My allowance was two serves of bread, a small amount of protein and salad with no added fat. Everyone else's plate had sausages, burgers, potato salad and other delicious homemade foods. Mine had a bread roll and a small hamburger patty with some lettuce and tomato. I wondered why I had to go without the food I loved so much. I was deprived of the only thing that made me feel good. Other kids wanted to know why I was eating a "special meal." I felt like a freak. I also felt jealous of the other girls and boys who could seemingly eat anything and not have to restrict their intake. They were all skinny. I went home after the party, made extra sandwiches and threw in a few cakes and lollies to make up for what I had missed out on. I was comforted. Food was the friend I always could depend on.

I stayed with Weight Watchers for about eight weeks. I lost some weight, but it didn't last. When I told my mum that I didn't want to go to Weight Watchers any more, she readily agreed. Once again, she could prove her affection by providing me with the food I loved. She did try to prevent me from eating high calorie foods, saying "You know you should be watching your weight" or "Do you really think you should eat that?" Oh yes, guilt got to me, so I began to sneak food. This was another way I learnt to use food to cope with my feelings and this time it covered the pain of the guilt. If no one was in the kitchen, I would sneak in and make a sandwich or cut some cake and always cover my tracks by saying I didn't eat lunch at school or I was especially hungry today. I was good at being sneaky. I was also good at being fussy, and convinced mum to buy me special food. That way, I always had my own stash.

Entering high school was especially painful. By this time I was significantly overweight, to the point that my uniform was the largest size available at the time and it was tight and uncomfortable. As a teenager, I soon learnt the "joys" of extreme dieting to combat binge eating. For some of those years I lost a lot of weight. I never felt a sense of peace though as I was constantly obsessed with food, what I ate, what I didn't eat, combining carbohydrates with protein, and fruit only days. Even at my thinnest, I still thought I was fat.

After high school I continued the war with myself. Until, at nineteen years of age, I fell pregnant with my first son. For the first time my life felt special and I felt at peace with food. Eight years later, when I was pregnant with my second son, I had the same feeling of peace with food. I ate when I was physically hungry, chose food for its nutritional value, didn't think about foods at other times, and continued to live my life without my food obsession. I actually did not gain weight during both pregnancies. The doctor said if I wasn't pregnant, I would have lost a great deal of weight! I could afford to stay the same weight while I was pregnant because I was overweight at the beginning of each pregnancy.

Once the boys were born, the war with food returned and I was well over one hundred kilograms within a few months of each birth. I hit my all time highest weight of one hundred and twelve kilograms, only three months after my second son was born.

During the years between the pregnancies I tried every diet imaginable. I went to Weight Watchers again, and each time I failed I would sign up at a new venue where no one would know me. I did this four times. Over the years I also tried Jenny Craig, Ultra Lite, meal replacement diets and various dieticians. I counted calories, fat and carbohydrates. I bought every new release diet book that was available. I had a subscription to *Slimming Magazine*. I knew everything there was to know about nutrition. But the food war persisted.

If you are reading this book then you have probably tried as many diets and counted as many calories as I have. You may also know the pain of looking at the scales and letting them determine whether you are going to have a great day or a depressing day. Are you able to count the number of times you have started a diet, program or other restricting food method? Think about the weight you have lost and gained. If you are anything like me the number of diets amount to more than you can count on two hands, not to mention the thousands of dollars paid out and hundreds of kilograms gained and lost. For me, the energy that this has consumed is incredible. I wonder what I would have been able to achieve if I had not spent all that time, energy and money on my war with food.

War …

My war continued and the more it continued, the more pain I felt. Every time I lost weight, I thought I was winning the war—but I was still in pain. The only way I knew to numb the pain was to eat, so I struggled with food and always gained weight back after a diet. It was a battle between dieting, breaking the diet, giving up, binging, and beating myself up.

It was a vicious cycle. It went round and round while I went crazy investigating the newest fad in dieting or signing up at the next Weight Watchers meeting.

I didn't understand the origin of my pain at the time. I believed that I was in pain because I was overweight. I thought if I could control my food intake, I could control my pain. So I put all my focus on my food. This seemed to work, in a strange sort of way. Eating numbed my painful feelings. Organising a diet or counting calories distracted me from my pain. As a result, all those unacknowledged feelings were buried deeper and deeper within the excess fat. Any time that I didn't have food as a focus, my real emotions started to surface. Fortunately, there was always more food to push them back down.

As long as I was busy fighting my war, I didn't have to think about the real reason I was eating. These reasons were so ingrained from a young age and I hadn't dealt with them for a long time. When I was a child and tried to acknowledge the feelings by talking to someone, I was pushed away. As soon as I would feel unsafe, anxious, worried, or even happy, food was an easy fix. Whether I was happy or sad, it seemed I had to even out my emotions. Eating until I was stuffed seemed to dull my feelings. If I felt happy, I ate to celebrate; if I felt sad, I ate to commiserate. Eating also provided an easy distraction. Instead of acknowledging my uncomfortable feelings, eating would numb them. I felt temporary comfort in the food. The quicker I ate, the quicker I felt the hole in the middle of my soul close over. Then to create further distraction from the real issue, I would hold my focus on how much I ate, how fat I felt and how I would resolve this by starting a new diet tomorrow or Monday or after the staff dinner on Friday. I felt like crap.

And Peace …

It was this cycle of dieting, binging, and feeling like crap, that made me realise that there had to something else to the problem of continually losing and gaining weight. Experiencing true peace with food during both pregnancies gave me some insight into what was going on. I occasionally had periods of true peace following my second pregnancy and started to recognise the pattern of my behaviour. When I was at peace, food became a secondary part of my life.

The first time I recognised this pattern and acknowledged my real physical hunger was in a fast food outlet. My real physical hunger was at three to four. (See *Insight to Peace 1.*) I definitely felt hungry for protein and I wanted a salad! My usual order at a fast food outlet was a burger and fries. I imagined what it would feel like if I ate the heavy greasy chips and the doughy white bread. I remember connecting with my hunger and asking myself what my body wanted. I wanted lightness in body, mind and soul. Somehow it didn't seem appealing and I ordered the burger without the chips and an orange juice. I ate slowly and mindfully, enjoying each bite.

The first result of my mindful eating experience was that the food did not cover up or push down feelings. Its main purpose was to nourish and fuel my body. This was a new experience for me and I felt physically and emotionally light. I felt completely satisfied after that meal. That was the start of a new way to think about the food I ate.

The second result of recognising the pattern was that I dealt with feelings as they arose, especially when the triggers were from the painful past. The first thing I did was acknowledge that I was physically hungry. If I wasn't physically hungry, then I needed to name the feeling and what I really wanted. This is how I got to where I am now. My insight was developing to a point where I would stop and understand whether it was real physical hunger I was feeling or something else. It was at these times that I naturally lost weight without dieting and was at peace with food.

Peaceful Food

Being at peace with food is glorious! I was once one hundred and twelve kilograms but when some peace was made, I lost around thirty kilograms without dieting. I also started to think about the nature of what I was really eating. Not the calories or the fat or the carbohydrates, but the "peacefulness" of the foods. For example, I have not eaten at any fast food outlets for years. I do not go to them and I do not take my children to them. I really thought about what this food was—fried, greasy, three week old chicken, more fried chips, no salad to be seen, and the most important thing—I was still hungry after I ate it! I also acknowledged how that food made me feel after I ate it. I felt lethargic and weighed down. There was a lump in my stomach when I finished. This food brought me no peace.

I knew there were foods that made my soul heavy. So I started to recognise that there were foods that made my soul sing! I knew I was onto something here. When I felt satisfied about the food I ate, the quality, its texture, its peacefulness, I felt less struggle with food.

How did I know what a peaceful food was? This seemed like such an important part of my journey. I didn't realise it but I was intuitively deciding what peaceful foods were by firstly avoiding fast food outlets and pre-packaged foods. When I look at pre-packaged food, I notice two things. Firstly, very few of its original ingredients are recognisable and secondly the "nutrition" label contains a whole lot of numbers that don't represent any fresh food that I know of! These numbers are added flavours, preservatives and other synthetic ingredients that make up for the lack of fresh and natural food. It feels to me as if these ingredients have been through a war themselves, before they ended up in the packet!

Here is a challenge for you. Bake a cake from a pre-packaged cake mix. Then make one from scratch, with real organic eggs, stone ground flour and real raw cacao powder. Compare the two, and tell me which one is a peaceful food.

Now I said earlier that this approach would have no diet plans, no counting calories, fat or carbs. Yes this is true! But knowing a food makes you feel good means it is a peaceful food. I believe a peaceful food should have the following qualities:

1. There is little or no processing—compare processed food and all those hostile ingredients with fresh, natural food.
2. You made it yourself so you are at peace with what's in it. No surprise attacks.

3. You can identify its core ingredients—they are recognisable by touch, smell and taste.

4. You are at peace with the nutrition label. If there are numbers listed, at least they have an explanation.

5. With fresh fruit and vegetables, you are at peace with the way they were grown, and the distance they have travelled. You know that they have been enriched by the local community.

6. It makes your soul sing! This includes the amount of food. You feel light, happy and energised at the end of the meal.

A food you love has the above qualities but first and foremost it makes you feel good. You can look at it and honestly say it is beautiful. You can imagine the farmer who grew it or the baker who baked it and you can feel gratitude for that person who provided you with this glorious food. My favourite chocolate is Lindt milk chocolate balls in the red wrapper. Not the blue wrapper, not the gold wrapper, and when I have chocolate this is the chocolate I usually choose. I want to taste every bite and I make it last. I am thankful to those Swiss Master Chocolatiers who have perfected the art of chocolate making. Why would I spend a second eating anything else?

Some other foods I love are avocado, fresh strawberries, rockmelon, watermelon, green seedless grapes, baby spinach, roast pumpkin (with the skin on!), barbequed calamari, freshly brewed organic coffee, Tasmanian feta cheese, vegetarian pizza with kalamata olives (homemade by me!), kettle-cooked potato chips and organic corn chips, and much more.

My list of foods I love has some common elements. They are fresh; they have little or no additives, preservatives, or numbers that I don't understand; I know where they come from; I trust the brand will give me the best quality possible. I can hear you saying already "What about the cost?" In fact, once you start eating peaceful food you love, your food bill drops significantly. No longer are you stocking the shopping basket with "fillers" that take up space and money, and rely on heavy energy production. You want the best and the best means you are honouring yourself with quality rather than quantity.

Start your own list of food you love based on the criteria above. It is easy to identify peaceful foods. Start with fresh foods. Which ones do you love to eat? Which do you know are local and organic? Think of all the chocolate you have eaten, which type makes your heart sing? Which type has quality above anything else? Which type makes your soul sing?

Love and peace, what a grand combination!

At Peace with the Journey

Although I have lost over twenty kilograms, I have found it difficult to continue the journey at times. After all, this is a journey, not a destination. We all know there are no quick fixes and this isn't one either. I have a long history of using food as a way to cope with feelings. The weight is not going to disappear overnight and this is not about perfection. I am writing this book so you can join me in this journey, witness my insights and help celebrate my progress. My quest for perfection fuels my war with food. When I diet, I set high standards for myself, and then fail. I punish myself further by binging and the cycle continues. Giving up dieting feels scary, as I have relied on it for so long. I know dieting doesn't work. Yet I continue to go on the diet/binge cycle. The promise of a diet—the promise of what it will achieve—is so seductive. I am never in the present with dieting, it is always future focussed, like finding the Holy Grail. I need a new way to approach this. I need to be at peace with the journey.

At Peace Dealing with Issues

Sometimes, when I eat food and I do not have real physical hunger, it feels like my soul is at war. This is part of the struggle. Recognising why I eat when I am not physically hungry is part of this journey. I have the most difficulty when my life is not as I want it to be. When I have lots of stress or I am in a difficult relationship or something happens that triggers emotion from the past I look to food first for comfort. These are the things that I still have to work with. I can find myself distracted by a diet or my weight or something else to do with my body, rather than focusing on the real issue. I know that I will feel at peace with myself once I have dealt with the real issue. Even better, I know that I can feel at peace with myself *while* I am dealing with these issues.

At Peace with the Media

I still get tricked sometimes into believing that the latest diet is a miracle diet. When I see the *Biggest Loser* on television or see a new article in a women's magazine, I want to find out more. I get sucked in to the advertising hype designed to sell readers or viewers. I have a simple solution to this one. I turn the TV off and I don't buy ANY women's magazines. The less influence that others have over my thinking the better.

The same goes for any new diet book. If you follow this simple approach you will never need another diet book again. Have you ever noticed that for every diet or food plan claiming the best diet, there is another claiming a better diet? If you really listen to your body, you will know what is best for you. You don't need to follow the hype. Of course, the only exception to this is if a doctor has advised that you must follow a particular diet for medical reasons. I have found that if you follow this simple approach you will naturally follow your doctor's advice anyway! You won't feel deprived because you are listening to your body. Your body knows what is best. When you listen to your body you are working with peace, when you don't you are struggling. I am at peace with the media. Are you?

At Peace with Perspective

I believe that you will lose weight when you recognise the food you eat, and why you are eating it. I believe that you will lose weight when you analyse your food—yes, analyse it! Not from a caloric or fat content perspective, but from the perspective of peace. There is no requirement for you to eat or not eat ANY food. You make the final decision. But now your decision will be made thoughtfully and with purpose. It will change the way you look at food and you will appreciate it for what it really is— fuel for your body. Why waste time and energy on cheap fuel that won't make you run efficiently? Why eat foods that make you sick and leave you needing a lot of fine-tuning in the future? I am at peace with my perspective. Are you?

At Peace with Being Yourself

I still panic about eating when I do not have real physical hunger, but now I address it differently. I ask myself "If you are not physically hungry then what are you really hungry for?" It is when you recognise and begin to deal with this that true peace with food will come. Acknowledging where you are now and that you have come a long way already is a big step. When you decide that you have had enough of diets, you will be ready to take your next step. A step that is life changing. Once you make the decision to get truly in touch with who you are and what you believe in, you will feel comfortable expressing your feelings without the need for food to push them back down. It is time to be at peace with being yourself.

At Peace with Exercise

Exercise is also part of making peace with food and your life. When you lead a full life, exercise comes naturally. I choose to walk every morning. It is my thinking time and it feels like a meditation for me.

I used to hate exercise and would do everything to avoid it. I would puff just walking up a flight of stairs, but now that I love life I prefer to walk up the stairs, have a little skip, go to the beach and walk along the water's edge, walk in the park, throw a football with the kids, dance in my lounge room (or on the dance floor!) and go for my morning walk. It is like I am breathing life into my body when my heart beats a little faster and I breathe a little more heavily. I love the feeling. I am also grateful that I can include this as part of my day. It doesn't have to be a big commitment or any commitment at all. Because as you become more peaceful with food the desire to exercise becomes more natural and it will be a regular inclusion in your life.

If you love the gym, then go for it! Personally, I don't like repetitive exercise. I love horse riding, playing tennis or squash, walking (anywhere!) and shooting hoops. This to me is fun and this is what exercise should be about in my eyes. If it is not fun it is not worth it. I am at peace with exercise. Are you?

The Good Stuff (and Bad)

I know when I make peace with food everything falls into place. I could not have maintained this thirty kilogram weight loss if I was still at war with my food.

I know that following this approach works. It is not about diet, deprivation or any other regulation of food intake. It is about identifying real physical hunger and eating the food you love from a peaceful perspective. Knowing that you are sick of the diet/binge cycle is enough to break free. Can you imagine a life where you have no emotional attachment to food, where you can look at it and feel gratitude for its presence, and its ability to provide sustenance to you in that moment? It is possible for the pleasure of food to play a minor part of your life instead of an all-consuming part. Start with the very next mouthful. Make it count. Here's how:

- ∾ Identify peaceful foods and the foods that you really love—your soul sings when you eat them.
- ∾ Recognise when you experience real physical hunger.
- ∾ If your hunger is not real physical hunger, identify and deal with feelings as they arise.
- ∾ Live a full life—and exercise will come naturally.

You will still struggle from time to time. When I am in this struggle, nothing else seems to matter.

I don't want to think about peaceful foods, any food will do! I know that it means something else is going on in my life and I need to address it if I truly want to be at peace with food. The two go together, peaceful foods and a peaceful mind. I can lose weight peacefully. I have done it. I have lived it. But how can I lose weight peacefully when "The Struggle" takes hold of me?

2

The Struggle

A
T THE AGE OF TWENTY-EIGHT, I weighed one
hundred and twelve kilograms. I lived with
a violent man. The only way I could escape
was by binge eating. I had been in my war with food
for many years. No wonder I felt depressed.

To understand my darkest hour I had to go back
to my childhood. It was not going to be easy but
it was where the struggle originated. My struggle
with food kept me from addressing the pain of my
childhood. Until I was able to recognise the reasons
why I ate in the first place I would always struggle.

Childhood Struggle

My mum says one of the reasons I was so fat as a
child is because Dad used to feed me the fat from

lamb chops. I love that story because it shows how mum made so many excuses for my weight. Funnily enough, I don't like lamb chops much. Mum cared for me, but couldn't recognise that my weight was about something much deeper. She saw that I ate too much, ate fatty foods and continued to gain weight.

I don't remember eating lamb chops as a child. I do remember two words my dad often said to me— "you're hopeless." He would arrive home from the pub late and intoxicated. His dinner would have gone cold, and mum would show her disgust by giving him the silent treatment. In response, Dad would pick on me. He'd find something I was hopeless at and begin to rant and rave. Mum would tell him to shut up, but to no avail. She tried to protect me from the harshness of his words. Dad continued his rave until he fell asleep in his chair at the dining room table. I wished I was somewhere else. I felt heartbroken, but tried very hard not to show any emotion. Once Dad fell asleep I could continue eating. Actually, I had been eating all afternoon. I had prepared myself for his abuse by binge eating since I arrived home from school.

I fell into the habit of eating all afternoon after school. I remember arriving home from school and making toast. This is one of the many memories of using food as a coping strategy. How many slices of toast did I make? I placed two slices of bread in the toaster not once, not twice, but five times. Ten slices of toast for an eight-year-old girl. Even now, I feel ashamed telling you how much food I ate. But it was easier for me to focus on food and self-blame than to recognise what was happening in my childhood. I felt so alone and unsupported.

My mother supported me in her own special way. She recognised that I was using food as a coping strategy and she encouraged that because she had a lot of difficulty showing her affection in other ways. It was very easy for her to say, "Come on darling, don't be upset, let's have some cake." Mum did not have an issue with food but she liked her sweets. She could eat just one piece of cake and be satisfied and find her peace with that. I could not because the first piece started to fill the void and so I thought I needed the second, third and fourth piece.

During those childhood years I learnt very succinctly how to numb any emotion with food in any situation. I was bullied by some other children who I thought were my friends. Their parents were friends of my mum and dad. One day they came over and all the kids went out into the back yard. I decided to jump on the clothesline and get the other kids to push me, just like a merry-go-round. I remember having so much fun and we were all laughing. My brother was also there and he was laughing. The two other boys were older. I was six, my brother was five and the two other boys were about ten and eleven. They thought it would be hilarious as I swung around to pull my pants down. They did it. They laughed and humiliated me and I felt deeply ashamed. The way I handled that incident that day had a significant impact my life. So what did I do? I ate. It was all I could do. When I ate I forgot the pain of that humiliation. I learnt to protect myself from getting hurt the only way I knew how. Eating protected me from uncomfortable feelings.

Those boys did not stop there. Every day I endured their torments at school. One day I was by the water taps with my friends. I saw the two boys coming. They were with their friends who were in a higher grade. I put my head down to the tap hoping they didn't see me. But they didn't miss any opportunity to humiliate me. "Hey fatty boom sticks!" they called. I recoiled, knowing they wouldn't stop. "Hey fatty boom sticks we're talking to you!" I walked away but they called out louder and followed me. They continued and all I could do was keep walking as fast as I could to get away. Every time I saw the boys at school they could not help themselves. They always called me names. If I saw them coming I would change direction, go the long way to my destination, or hide in the toilets until they had moved on. After that first time many of the other kids at the school also called me names. The more it happened the more I came home and ate. I remember mentioning the bullying to my mother, and she acknowledged there was a problem, but nothing much changed. My mum didn't talk to the boys' mum much at all after that. Mum told me not to worry, just ignore any name calling, it'll be alright. But I began putting up a barrier, and that was the protective physical barrier of fat.

Teenage Struggle

From my childhood experiences I learnt that when horrible feelings surfaced, eating provided comfort. Eating numbed me; I focussed on my food, rather than my problems. Because I was stuffing down so many bad feelings, being overweight became an obvious issue. As I mentioned earlier, I first attended Weight Watchers when I was ten years old. I thought I was doing something wrong by eating too much. Then I reached high school. I learned that by eating less and making myself attractive, I could encourage boys to take some interest in me.

As a teenager my war with food continued, but I had a new ally—peer pressure. My friends and

I talked about makeup, clothes and boys. I had learned in primary school that boys are scary; they can hurt and humiliate you. What better time to extreme diet than as a teenager? I had the support of my peers and we all believed that losing weight was highly desirable. The focus changed from what I ate to what I didn't eat. I had one friend in particular who was my best source of support. We fought our war with food together. We would eat fruit for days then have a steak and potato on Friday night. We both lost a lot of weight. We constantly talked about what we could and couldn't eat. Some days we ate nothing but watermelon and we couldn't wait until Friday night for our steak and potato. The name-calling stopped as I was no longer fat, but I still felt insecure. I used my dieting to distract me from the real emotional issues. If I broke the diet I felt more self-hatred and despair. I would immediately resolve to be even stricter with myself the next day.

My dad still thought I was hopeless, and told me so. My extreme diet gave me the confidence to ignore him, or call him names. I focussed on my diet, rather than his harsh words. My mum resisted my diet at first, saying I shouldn't be so strict on myself, but as time went by she loved buying me "special food" and preparing special meals. She could easily show me in her own way how much she loved me.

I felt like a coiled spring, pushed tighter and tighter with extreme dieting. Eventually, after leaving high school I abandoned the world of extreme dieting to return to the world of binge eating. I quickly piled on weight. At eighteen I was around one hundred kilograms.

Adult Struggle

As an adult I decided that my weight problem was this horrible thing that I was doing to my body. I was making this happen because I was greedy, eating the wrong foods, and not eating healthily. It was all about food. The more I focused on what I was or wasn't eating and losing weight, the bigger the problem grew.

It is only now in hindsight that I recognise the feelings I was trying to avoid. I felt like I was "emotionally gutted", a feeling so uncomfortable that only food covered the emptiness. The emptiness had to be filled one way or another by constant eating or obsessing about food. I always avoided feeling empty. I started to panic if I thought I would miss a meal. I felt vulnerable. So I filled the emptiness with something else, either food or thinking about food. I needed fullness, not emptiness.

It was the fullness of life that was missing and I used food to create it. When I used food it changed my energy. Being full made me lethargic. When I was weighed down it gave me an excuse not to address my feelings but to focus on where the fullness originated—from food.

My darkest period was from twenty-six to thirty-one years of age. I lived with Bill, and he too was at war with food. Neither of us would have said we had a problem at the time. He was a violent man from a violent childhood. Violence equals abuse, and abuse comes in all different forms. We had both experienced different forms of abuse in our childhood so we found an instant connection. Only now when I look back do I realise what it was that bound us together. Food was our bond.

When two souls in denial join together they compound each other's food obsession. One day we were sitting at home watching TV and we decided to go and get some fast food. Of course, this meant a visit to the drive-thru then returning home and watching more TV. So we went to the fast food outlet and ordered up big. It was usual to order the largest size. I can't ever remember when I had ordered a small size. So we ate our food but this time the food wasn't enough and an argument started. Bill punched me in the face. I remember calling the police, and him running away. I stayed at Mum and Dad's place that night; the next day, I went back to him.

Mum knew about Bill's violence. If I would mention it she would say, "Well there are good things about him, he cleans the house well." The fact that he could vacuum somehow overrode the physical pain I endured. My mum and I talked over a cup of tea and cake. We never talked about the details of what actually happened. Nor did we ever talk about what happened when I was a child. The way Mum helped me to ease my feelings was by preparing a special meal or special food.

When I was in denial about my true feelings I ate more and more. I didn't think I was any good for anyone. I had been brainwashed into believing that I was helpless and hopeless. I believed that I couldn't possibly do any better than Bill. If I acknowledged all the negative experiences in my life, the pain would be too great for me to bear. It would feel like dying. So it was easier to eat the food and forget about those experiences. I could then focus on my weight and my diet plans, rather than facing the reality of my bad relationship. Food was very seductive. It took me away from the real issues very quickly.

Lessening Struggle

It took two major crises for me to leave Bill once and for all. The first was Bill's major violent outburst. The second was my mum's diagnosis of terminal cancer.

As soon as I left the relationship, my war with food died down. I gained some insight into the true cause of my feelings of emptiness, and lost ten kilograms very quickly. I started to tune in to my body and really listened to what it was telling me. I noticed sometimes there was emptiness, but it wasn't real physical hunger. It was something else. I became curious about it, explored it and named it. I called it my "emotionally gutted" feeling. The "emotionally gutted" feeling originated from the area around my stomach and just below my navel. So now I knew that this was not real physical hunger.

Each time I became aware of this feeling I questioned my need for food. I found that food wasn't what I needed. I needed nurturing, security or love. I discovered the areas around my stomach and below my navel are related to chakras. A chakra is an energy centre dwelling in the body. There are seven basic chakras within our bodies.

- ∾ The root chakra at the base of the spine.
- ∾ The sacral chakra in the lower abdomen about two and half centimetres from the naval.
- ∾ The solar plexus chakra about halfway between the navel and base of the sternum.

- ⌘ The heart chakra in the centre of the chest.
- ⌘ The throat chakra in the middle of the throat.
- ⌘ The third eye chakra between the eyebrows.
- ⌘ The crown chakra at the centre on top of the head.

I felt "emotionally gutted" in my solar plexus chakra and sacral chakra. These are the two chakras closest to the stomach. I started to see the relationship between my body shape, and these chakras. My emptiness was in the middle of my body and most of my fat was distributed in the middle of my body. It seemed that the fat protected me where I needed it the most. Most women have weight around their root chakra (hips and thighs). Where do you have the highest fat distribution? Do you see a relationship between your fat distribution and the location of the chakras? What are your feelings about this? Gutted? Empty? Ungrounded? Unprotected? Or something else? I will explore the chakras further in a later chapter.

In my struggle with food I never felt full or satisfied. It was not about the food, it was about my dissatisfaction with life. By spending all my time, money and energy looking for the right diet meant less time for looking at the real issue and for finding something else that satisfied me in healthy ways. The spiral of looking, finding, trying, and failing took up all my thinking, time and energy. I was exhausted from the food obsession. Once I changed my focus, weight loss became a by-product of getting in touch with myself. What was your relationship with food as a child? What is your relationship with food now?

It was easy to deny my struggle, so how did I know when I was in it? Physically, I felt anxious and jittery—like a drug addict hanging out for a fix. As a child, every time I saw those boys at school, my body would tighten, and I would feel my gut preparing for battle. I avoided eye contact, and focussed on other things. But when they attacked me, the emotions built up inside. I wanted to scream at them. I wonder what would have happened if I had screamed, "Just leave me alone!" Would it have made a difference to the way I felt if I expressed my feelings? I didn't have a voice. If I had felt grounded and valued by others, I could have expressed my feelings. When I got home Mum said, "Just ignore them," but the pain was too intense and I didn't know how to cope. Mum had good intentions. I know now I felt gutted and my coping strategy was to eat.

So the pattern repeats over and over. Sometimes feelings come up and I still haven't learnt how to deal with them in a healthy way. I haven't learned how to nurture myself, and give myself permission to say, "I am allowed to feel." When I refuse myself permission to feel, I have to substitute with something else. I can binge, or I can obsess about the number of calories I am eating. And when I fail, when I break my self-imposed rules, I can punish myself. I can say, "Jen, you idiot! You are putting on weight, you are so fat!"

But if I punish myself, I am simply perpetuating the cycle of self-abuse. Now, I have another alternative. I can look into this further and ask myself, "What is missing in my life that I have to fill with food? What do I need right now?" This is what led me to tell my story and write this book. I needed to be heard. I want women to understand there is more to life than diets and obsessing about food. I want women to feel they are not alone, because that is how I felt—alone.

I was attracted to junk food because they offer a quick fix. They are able to change my mood within minutes. Even simple food such as bread can be addictive. White bread is a good example. It is a processed product with lots of additives and refined ingredients such as white flour and sugar. It was very easy for me to eat lots of slices of white bread and not feel full. When I eat good quality bread such as organic spelt wholegrain bread it is more difficult to eat to excess, because it is so filling. In the past I would have thought that I wasn't worth spending the extra money on an organic spelt loaf of bread. When you feel physically hungry, it's best to eat high quality food. And if you feel emotionally hungry, affirm your self-worth by feeding yourself high quality food. High quality food is the best solution if you choose to eat for both types of hunger. For example, my favourite breakfast food is toast—organic spelt bread, avocado and squeeze of lemon. The bread label lists the following ingredients: organic wholegrain spelt flour including a number of other organic flours, sesame and poppy seeds. The grains are grown in Australia, and the bread is baked locally.

So by choosing this food I am honouring my self-worth. Yes, it is more expensive than a basic white bread, but I can look at every ingredient and truly know that the bread was made for my health and nutrition. This food is high quality fuel. I know that I will feel good after eating it. I feel light and I am full of useable energy. In a later chapter I will discuss this idea in more detail. You do not have to exclude any food, but most importantly nor do you have to eat to stuff down your negative feelings.

What happens if you think there is no issue causing your negative feelings? That all that really matters is food and diet? You may prefer to believe that everything else in your life is great except for the diet. Look further into yourself. Is there pain? Are you sick of the constant obsession with food and diets? Have you had a long history of diets, losing weight, and gaining weight? If you thought it was only about diet, you would have chosen the latest diet book, instead of a book about peace. There is a war and you feel it. Now it is time to find out why. You may know that something is there but you can't see it yet. Recognising your inner struggle allows you to take next step. You can move on from here.

Present Day Struggle

While writing this chapter, something happened. I started eating. At first it was because I had a real physical hunger, but that wasn't enough. I looked for more. My partner had some fun size chocolates in the downstairs fridge. I ate five, and I ended up with a headache. I was not at peace. I had two choices—beat myself up or be curious. I have learnt to embrace the struggle. It tells me that something is not right. I can use food to prepare for perceived pain or deal with emotional pain. I can also use food as a reason to celebrate. I don't have to make excuses to eat food. Food is socially acceptable. From the outside, everyone sees your life as great— loving partner, happy kids, and a comfortable house. Events that happened so long ago in childhood are easy to forget. But these patterns are deeply ingrained. They are easily triggered when someone judges or criticises me. When someone triggers similar feelings by using judgement, criticism, or harshness I prepare myself for the perceived pain that may follow. Talking with my brother triggers uncomfortable feelings. I was at a barbeque recently where my brother attended. At first I was at peace with food. I ate because I had real physical hunger. Then as time went on I noticed I was picking at foods, eating more than I needed. The conversation had turned to what my dad was doing. It alerted me that some emotions had been stirred up. Something else was going on. I became aware and I was able to refocus my intention for being at the barbeque, and enjoying the company of others.

It has been important for me to understand that I use my struggle to obsess about food and diet rather than reflecting upon my emotional state. When I hear myself say, "I wonder how many calories in this food" or "I shouldn't eat this," I know that food is distracting me from other issues. I began to understand what was going on when I became curious about my behaviour. This transformed my struggle. I call it "walk the bridge and just get over it." I do this by not buying into any conversations (with myself or others) about food and what I should or shouldn't eat. I look beyond the food for answers. I ask myself, "What is going for me right now?" I show myself some compassion by doing something non-food related. I go for a walk, read a good book, or put on some essential oils. I do something for me.

The answer is not to exclude food but to find peace with food. The more that I work with this the less I struggle. I am better able to walk the bridge and get over it. The more I investigate my feelings and learn from them, the further I am able to move on without judgement. I can take the opportunity to embrace this learning or I can go back to the war with food. I don't want to go back to the war with food. Being grounded is the first step to addressing, maybe even transforming the struggle. I didn't understand how it felt to be centred and grounded for a long time. Now it is the basis for understanding my war with food. All I need to learn now is to transform the struggle, so I can be my real self and lose weight easily. So how do I move towards transforming the struggle?

3

Transforming Struggle

*T*HIS FEELS GOOD. Something has changed in me. "The Struggle" has been transformed. I know I do not need to struggle anymore. It feels like walking across a bridge to a new land. I know how far I have come and that I could pause, and look back, but I keep moving forward. I want to get to the other side.

The other side is similar, but different. I can look at my experiences with new eyes. All the emotional pain I have experienced has taught me new ways to handle my feelings. Knowing how far I have travelled gives me the confidence I need to keep going.

I call this process "transforming struggle". It is the struggle that has led to these positive changes.

I used to think I was a food addict or compulsive eater, but now I realise it isn't true. Have you heard of "trigger foods"? Once you begin eating a trigger food, you can't stop. One bite is all it takes. The food that triggers a binge is usually a high fat, high calorie junk food. Pizza, for example, is a classic example of a trigger food. I have often read that compulsive eaters and food addicts should "stay away from trigger foods" if they want to lose weight. But there are days when I can eat a whole pizza and still feel empty, while there are other days when I can eat two slices of pizza and feel totally satisfied. Being a food addict doesn't explain why this happens.

What is the difference? Why do some pizzas leave me feeling hungry, while others satisfy me completely? It all depends upon the quality of the pizza. If I order a fast food chain pizza with a thick crust and a high-fat topping, the chances are that I'll scoff the lot. On the other hand, if I order from our locally run pizza restaurant, I take my time, enjoy the experience and appreciate the skills of the Australian-Italian chef who prepared it. I know he makes his pizzas with love and passion. He loves to cook for customers who appreciate his artistry. Compare this to a production line operation where pizzas are rushed through to satisfy the bulk orders coming in.

This example has shown me that it is possible to think differently about food. When I buy from my local pizzeria, I think differently. I come to the meal with a different mindset. This is my peace. It is not only peace with food but peace with life. I approach my meal in the spirit of gratitude and serenity. I know that my actions have consequences. I know that I deserve the quality that only my local Australian-Italian chef can provide for me. I know that his heart and soul are in his restaurant. I honour him with my patronage, and he honours me with the meal he serves.

But I hear you say, "I love those chain store pizzas!" Yes I THOUGHT I did until I compared the experience. When I order a chain store pizza, I scrounge around for a current discount voucher. I know I would feel cheated if I had to pay full price. When the pizza arrives, I devour it quickly. It's not food, but fuel, and poor quality fuel at that. This is not peaceful eating. Even after I have satisfied my hunger I want to keep eating. Chain store pizzas are made to fill you up. Check out the thickness of the crust compared to the topping. Really look at your pizza and use *Insight into Peace 2* to see if it is really the food you love. Find your peace with pizza!

So how did I come to realise that a transformation was occurring? In the previous chapter I introduced the chakras—energy centres dwelling in the body. I came to this understanding through meditation.

Once I was centred and grounded (see *Insight into Peace 14*) I visualised the chakras and the energy stuck within them. I asked myself which parts of my body have emotional blocks. I began to understand why I eat when I don't have real physical hunger. I tuned into my body and its needs. I honoured what my body was telling me. If I sensed that some energy was stuck, I could explore this further, without eating to cover it up. To do this further, I wrote down the feelings associated with this stuck energy. One of my favourite exercises was to pretend that this energy could tell me the reason why it was stuck. I would listen to this energy, and write down what it told me. I slowly became aware of my feelings, and with that awareness came peace. It did take some practice but I continued to do it more and more each day until it felt like the natural way to respond to an uncomfortable feeling.

To help release the stuck energy, I also used therapeutic grade essential oils (see *Appendix*). Essential oils help me to connect with myself on a new level. When I breathe in their aromas, they access the limbic system of the brain. The limbic system is where memories and trauma are stored. Essential oils may stimulate the areas of the brain associated with memory and learning. They may influence hormonal responses, and they can also alter moods and feelings. My favourite way to use the oils is to place one drop on my hand then massage it onto my body, particularly on the chakras. I hold the energy by keeping my hand in place until I feel a shift occur. Sometimes this will be a thought or a feeling, a sensation in my body or just a deep sense of relaxation.

I didn't have to go around meditating with my hands in a prayer position twenty-four hours a day to tune into my body's needs. But I did gain a general feeling of wellbeing. When something went wrong, I knew it was not the end of the world, and I didn't have to eat to make it better. I was learning a new way to live and a new way to love myself. The benefit was that I was losing weight without the obsession with dieting and food.

Exploring the Transformation

I had been at war with food for many years, so I could not expect the transformation to lead to instant change. It took many realisations about who I was and how I got here. The fat was an obvious sign of my struggle, and coming to terms with that was difficult. It wasn't about dieting, losing weight or counting calories. It was about using food as a coping strategy for just about everything that came my way. Food made me tired, heavy and overweight.

It was my excuse for not participating in life. Want to go for a walk? No thanks, I'm too puffed. Take the kids to the park? Sorry, I'm too tired. It was easy to opt out and say it was all too much trouble. I was so unhappy that I didn't have anything to look forward to—except food.

After my relationship with Bill ended, I lost ten kilograms. This was my first insight into how my life was changing. The rest of the weight took some years to come off, but it always happened when I was aware of my feelings, when I acknowledged what was going on in my life. You will be able to gather the insights that took me years to discover and use them to transform your life now. This approach is miraculous: when you discover how much life means to you, you will lose weight just by being at peace with yourself. You won't have to worry about weight or food.

What it Means for the Past (Seeing Things Differently)

When you have experienced childhood trauma, it is sometimes easy to ignore the past—or to remain stuck there. In my case, childhood trauma gave me the excuse I needed to avoid looking at myself. I refused to look into the psychological reasons behind my war with food. You may find that as issues come up, you need professional counselling. Please seek the help of a professional counsellor if you feel that you are stuck or not able to cope with the emotions you are feeling.

Many years of binging and dieting created the illusion that my struggle was about food. My experiences make me the person I am. I needed to reach my lowest point before I gained my insight. I was being taught a lesson that I had to learn. Sometimes I didn't learn the lesson at first, so it took years of struggle to finally change my thinking. Change occurs when we take notice of the lesson, and use this new information in a different way.

One of the first lessons I learnt was crucial. I found by acknowledging the impulses that drove me to eat as a child allowed me to make peace with them. I dealt with the shame of being bullied and put down by eating, and this became my way of coping with negative feelings.

I also learnt that I needed to forgive myself. For years, I had blamed myself for being overweight. I blamed myself because I believed I should have been able to control my eating. Sometimes, I managed to lose weight, but then the weight came back, more than ever. This signalled to me that I had not dealt with the underlying issues. My body was telling me that unless I dealt with these issues, I would continue to put on weight. I felt a sense of urgency. The more I ate, the more weight I gained, and the more desperate I became. Sometimes it means exploring things that may not be immediately apparent. I had to look deep into my past to find the answers.

I needed to forgive those family members who had hurt me. You might be wondering why I would need to forgive my father for treating me the way he did. After all, he did the best he could while dealing with his own pain. He behaved the way he did for good reasons, even if I could not fathom them. His experiences, whatever they were, made him the parent that he was. My experiences made me the person I am today. They have given me the insight to be able to say, "I love my dad for who he is." It doesn't mean that I would allow him to treat me badly today. But as an adult I choose when I want to see him, and I choose how I interact with him. Most of all, I have gained insight into how his comments affected me.

This insight also helped me to acknowledge the continuing patterns that I had carried into adulthood. For example, there was a time when I could not have imagined forgiving Bill for his behaviour. But today I see him for what he truly is—a person who hasn't dealt with his demons. He is still carrying them with him, right up to this day.

It doesn't help me to begrudge the years that I chose to stay with him in a violent relationship. I have to take responsibility for my part of the relationship. I allowed the cycle of violence to continue because I thought I didn't deserve any better. Now I speak up for myself if I feel that someone's actions are inappropriate.

I choose the company of people who treat me the way I deserve to be treated.

I see my childhood tormentors differently, too. I remember swinging on the clothesline as a child, and imagine that I can stand up for myself. When the boys attack me I tell them that they are immature. I send them home; I won't be their friend if they treat me that way. When I'm walking through the playground at school the boys call me bad names. "Leave me alone," I reply. "I am telling the teacher." And then they leave me alone.

I know that I am re-imagining my personal history. Those boys hurt me deeply. But it is important for me to help my inner child feel safe again. And we all have an inner child that wants to feel safe and cared for. Being grounded and centred is a good way to do that. Our inner child possesses an innate spontaneity. It responds to the world with curiousness, sensitivity, and wonderment. It feels alive. Those unhappy events of childhood stop us from expressing our inner child, because we feel unsafe. It does not matter if our fear is real, or only perceived. We must learn to nurture our inner child rather than criticise it.

Nurturing our inner child means making it feel safe, then allowing ourselves to express our feelings of joy. Have you ever wanted to scream at the top of your lungs or roll around on the ground laughing? You can do this! First, create a safe environment. You may want to scream into a pillow, or you might find a beautiful and private grassy area where you can roll around.

We need to allow ourselves enough time for the feelings to emerge. By allowing ourselves the time and safety we need to connect with our joy, we are saying we are worth it.

When we acknowledge our past and move towards forgiveness, when we allow ourselves to experience the joy in our lives, we start to have different priorities. By seeing things differently, food and dieting become less important.

Who am I Now?

The transformation is almost complete. I am here now, and I decide in every second who I will be. Will I be the scared child who cannot stand up for herself? Or will I be the fun, spontaneous child

who knows that she is safe to do whatever she wants? Right now, I allow that child to blossom within me.

I can do this by having fun! Before the pain of childhood there lived a child who could do anything with no fear of put downs, hurtful actions or comments. Living without fear is the best way to have fun. We can access our inner child to have fun too. Imagine you could do whatever you wanted right now—laugh until you cry, roll around in the grass at the park, dance to music in your lounge room. Just imagine how it would feel. Then choose something that gives you the same feeling. Watch a classic movie, go for a walk or dance in your lounge room!

If we listen to our inner child it will have something to say. It will be able to tell us what it needs right now. Sometimes we feel we are breaking the rules by allowing our inner child to have its say. If it has its say it will feel heard, safe and secure, and that is what I want for my inner child now. The child no longer has to feel scared and alone. The inner child is part of me that wants to feel safe.

I nurture the part of me that feels the pain of the past. But I nurture it in healthy ways, such as going for a walk in nature, writing or drawing to express my emotions, or speaking with a close friend. This allows me to express feelings that normally would be stuffed down or numbed with food. It is very important to acknowledge these feelings because they make me who I am. Without these experiences I could not have had the insights that I have around eating peacefully. So I am able to live in the now as a confident, happier and lighter person.

Being in the now allows me to move on. If I dwell in the past I spend all my time and energy there. That can be draining. I acknowledge the past but I am here now! My experiences have made me who I am. I acknowledge, forgive and live with the decisions I have made.

Transforming Shape

Part of transforming struggle is the transformation of my physical shape. Weight loss is the side effect of dealing with the pain that drove me to eat in the first place. When I was in my war with food, no matter how much weight I gained or lost I wore the same size clothes. As a teenager I remember wearing extremely baggy pants with a belt to keep them up. I had a pin holding my school uniform together at the waist. I wore oversize jumpers and loose tops. I did not accept myself for who I was. I thought I didn't deserve new clothes and certainly not in a smaller size.

My fat was my armour and when my armour wasn't physically present then the clothes were still bulky and protective. When my transformation became evident part of that was to honour myself and wear clothes that fitted properly. This meant going through my cupboard and removing anything that was too big or small. I didn't throw them away. Some I sold at online auctions, others I gave to friends and the rest I donated to charity. This is an exciting step to take. It reinforces the thought that "I am good enough."

At the time it meant that I had just a few clothes left. Second hand shops are one of the best places to buy "new" clothes. Now when I buy clothes if they don't fit me, I don't buy them. Accept yourself for who you are today. This is the beginning of the physical transformation.

Start this process by clearing your space. Set aside some time to try on every piece of clothing. Decide if it is the right size, colour and style for your body shape. If it is not right for you it is time to let it go. What does that piece of clothing give you? Is it your security for when you put weight on again? Is it your image of perfection that is too small? Does it hold a dream? Instead of focussing on what might be focus on what is here and now. Some of the smaller clothes you may choose to pack away but make sure they are out of your cupboard so that every day you can look at your cupboard and say "My clothes fit me perfectly in every way." By doing this you are affirming that you are okay right now.

Embracing "The Now"

We can allow things to happen and then we can let go. Letting go is part of forgiveness. We have to let go to embrace. It sounds like a contradiction in terms but what we let go and what we embrace are two different things. The old expression "forgive and forget" doesn't work for me. I say, "forgive and embrace." We forgive the past and the people but we embrace the lesson we learned. When we experience that pattern again we remember what we learnt and change the way we react to the situation.

Here is an example: One of the times that used to be most difficult for me was when I arrived home from work in the afternoon. I felt the urge to go straight to the kitchen. On reflection I saw that it was the time when I used to get home from school. The stresses of the day had built up and I needed the food to calm down. This was a lifelong pattern which began when I was bullied at school. When I arrived home I found comfort in food. I then used more food to prepare for my father's criticism that night.

By embracing these lessons now, I am able to move on from the past. I have come to understand why I behave the way I do. I can continue to live with the same pattern or I can choose to do things differently. Now when I come home from work I take the dog for a walk, chat with my partner or do some writing. I focus on how I am feeling right now. I acknowledge those feelings. What is your now? Is your now weighed down by the guilt of the past, or has it been liberated from the past? Take a minute to stop and observe *what you are thinking*. When we are caught up in our own story it stops us from moving forward. It is easier to blame than to take responsibility for our own actions. I can focus on my childhood trauma, my former abusive partner, or I can choose to move forward. When I made this decision it changed my life.

You may be wondering why you would want to embrace "the now." Perhaps you are too busy for all that nonsense. Perhaps you can't forgive the past; perhaps you don't even want to forgive. The decision to embrace the now must come from your heart. It will not work unless you take an honest look at where you have been, acknowledge it and then move on. To acknowledge the past you must let the feelings surface without using food to stuff them back down. What is the worst thing that could happen? The worst thing that could happen is that you will feel the pain of the past. It is time to stop being afraid of the pain and name it. What is the real identity of your pain? When the feelings come up, say something like "Hello Judgement, I see you are here today." Once you have acknowledged its presence, it is time to let it go. To let it go, practice the *Insights into Peace* in Chapter 8 which relate to feelings.

Here is the choice. If you avoid living in the now you will continue to use food, dieting, and binging as your focus. If you choose to be open and let yourself express your feelings you can move forward. Life can be what you want it to be. Living a life you never expected will make it brighter than ever. Can you make the decision to take the next step?

Diet to Peace

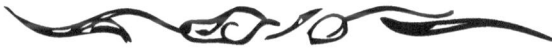

4

Make the Decision

I LOVE HOW MY LIFE HAS CHANGED. Since learning the art of peaceful eating, I have started to see my life from a different perspective. I have married my soul mate, and I quit my job after twelve years working in education. I see opportunities everywhere. Just writing this book demonstrates my ability to move forward without fear. Now I love taking those healthy risks that are part of living a full life. Before, I only felt content when I was in my food comfort zone.

I now have a plan for the future. It is not a plan based on wishful thinking. It is a real plan with real goals. Food is no longer the focus of my day. What would you think about if you didn't have to think about your next diet or your next binge? If you didn't think about food, what would take up the space? I will tell you. It is life! I started to make a life for myself.

Of course, before this, I also had a life, don't get me wrong. I went to university, I earned a Degree and a Master's Degree. But all that time I was not living my passion. I was trying to prove that I wasn't stupid. Thin people often assume that fat people are dumb. I had to prove them wrong. I also thought that academic success would compensate for those other areas of my life, such as relationships, which were so volatile. So I studied and I continued to study in an area that did not truly interest me. I loved helping people but I needed something else, and it wasn't until I learned the art of peaceful eating that this came to me.

The Secret

The most important step I took was to make the decision that things would be different. I couldn't continue the way I was. A typical day in the past went like this:

∾ The alarm goes off. I roll over, refusing to get out of bed. I linger for fifteen minutes or so until I can't leave it any longer or I will be late.

๛ I rush down my breakfast without a thought. I eat the same thing each morning—toast with lots of cheese. I already weigh myself down with food because I hate having to work in a job that is burning me out.

๛ I drive to work with tears in my eyes. There has to be a better way to earn a living.

๛ Once I arrive at work, I am immediately bombarded with extra tasks. There is no time for a break or time to prepare the food I am really hungry for. There is no time to honour my physical hunger. I eat at my desk when I have a spare minute or two. I stuff it down.

๛ Once I arrive home I make up for the food I missed during the day. Because my stress levels have built up so much I think I need food to calm me down. I continue to eat until I have pushed those uncomfortable feelings aside. Then I worry about how much food I have eaten and beat myself up until it is time to prepare dinner.

๛ I prepare dinner, not allowing myself the time I need to process the emotions

and stress I experienced during the day. I
feel resentful that I am the only member
of the house who is expected to prepare
food for everyone else.

∾ I prepare their favourite food. I don't
particularly like this food because it is
easy, fast, lacks care and quality.

∾ After dinner, I watch television. Once the
kids are in bed, I get out the chocolate so
I can really "relax."

∾ I go to bed with an uncomfortably full
stomach and thoughts of self-hatred. Why
did I eat so much? Why have I caused
myself so much pain?

∾ The next day the alarm goes off and it
starts all over again.

I know I have come so far. My decision to change
meant that I had to change my mindset.
My typical day now goes like this:

∾ I usually wake just before the alarm,
listen to a few songs, then turn the
alarm off. I review my plans for the day,
envisioning all the positive interactions
I will experience. I know that these
interactions will fill my life with joy and

abundance. I feel a surge of energy and gratitude.

∾ I rise, and go for a half-an-hour walk. It's time to wake up, see what is happening in the world first thing in the morning, and to clear my thinking for the day ahead. Also, this is when I feel most inspired. I can dream as much as I want while I'm awake!

∾ If I have real physical hunger I will eat breakfast once I am home, but usually I will fit in a few other things first. Usually, I don't eat until I am hungry. If I have to go out and I have no real physical hunger, I will eat something just so I don't become hungry at an inconvenient time. Sometimes I have to plan my meals based on my activities, and that is okay.

∾ My work day is varied now. I have chosen to run my own business. I enjoy every appointment, meeting and interaction I have.

∾ In the afternoon, I may take the dog for a walk, work on a project, or chat with my partner and son. Alternatively, I may give myself the space I need to reflect on the day's events.

∾ I prepare dinner thoughtfully. I don't
compromise on great taste or quality. The
food is fresh, organic and full of variety.
∾ After dinner I may watch some television,
but I also have activities I attend, such as
aromatherapy classes or the local women's
group activities.

My secret is that I decided that things would
be different in my life. But how did that decision
manifest itself in my behaviour? Firstly, I know that
something is not quite right when I am binge eating,
focussing on my diet or obsessing about food. I need
to identify the source of the problem before I can
make any changes. For me, I had to extract myself
from a violent relationship, change jobs and learn
gratitude for what I did have. My focus completely
changed. I didn't waste my energy on the next diet
or the food I was about to binge on. I developed
a clear intention for my life—to find peacefulness
within myself. I didn't meditate for hours on end or
constantly use affirmations. Instead, I established
some good old-fashioned goals for myself.

When I decided that things had to be different,
I wrote down the details of every aspect of my
life. Relationships, Career, Family, and Self. Then
I thought about what I really wanted in my life.

I imagined I had all the money in the world and I could do anything or have anything I wanted. I imagined where I would be, with whom I would live, how I would look and how I would be acting. I imagined it as if it had already happened.

Just because I made huge changes in my life doesn't mean that your changes have to be as dramatic. I made small changes first—creating time to go for a walk each day, making it to my son's sports carnival and watching his events, and taking a short course in aromatherapy. These small decisions led onto bigger goals. For example, my short course in aromatherapy inspired me to study for an Advanced Diploma in Aromatic Medicine. I found my passion and it shines through into all other aspects of my life. It also shines through in the goals I have set for the future.

Here's how you can identify your priorities in life. Find a note pad, or maybe even buy a special journal. An ordinary notepad will do the job, or you might want to buy a beautiful notebook with an embossed cover. But a fancy book can inhibit some people. They don't want to mess it up by roughing out their ideas. Once you have your journal, draw up a list. Describe your typical day as it is now. Then describe how you would like it to be. What are the differences between the two? Next, highlight what is important in the areas of relationships, career, family and self. Write down a goal for each area of your life, including a date by which you intend to achieve your goal. Two years ago I wrote this career goal: "To have my first book published by December 2009." At the time I had no idea how this would happen but I knew in my heart it was something I was passionate about. And now you are reading my dream! It was important for me to have my goal written down so that I could look at it, make it concrete and make it reality.

Taking some positive steps helped me to move my decisions into reality. The same will work for you. You don't have to take big steps. Writing down the details of my life helped me understand why I had made some poor decisions in the past. I didn't just arrive in a violent relationship because I was unlucky. I attracted the violent relationship because I was willing to accept his behaviour. I accepted it because I did not believe that I deserved to be treated well. Of course, my experiences earlier in life had helped make me feel hopeless. I was brought up to believe I was hopeless, so why would I expect to be treated well? As a result, I allowed people to treat me poorly. I played out that scenario in all my previous relationships as I was always treated second best.

I had to acknowledge that I felt hopeless. This was challenging, because it meant that I had to take responsibility for the life I had created for myself. The choices I made and the beliefs I adopted had all contributed to this. Only by acknowledging the reasons for my hopelessness could I truly understand my pain. Sometimes it is hard to break away from a relationship or career. Just acknowledging that a relationship or a career no longer serves you can be enough to move you forward. You can learn more from this acknowledgement. We tend to stay in a difficult relationship or job until we have learnt all that it can teach us. So don't beat yourself up by starting another binge or diet. Instead, look at your life. Ask yourself, "What is going on?" When you binge or diet, what emotions are you trying to cover up?

I didn't binge because I was greedy. Binging helped me hide from the real issues in my life: the pain of parental neglect, childhood bullying and a violent relationship. Binging comforted me. It was easy. Food was available anytime, anywhere, anyplace.

I finally saw there was a cycle. I felt the pain, but instead of acknowledging the pain, I ate, and the pain diminished. Then I beat myself up about eating, totally ignoring the real issue. Most times I acted unconsciously—until I noticed the cycle. Getting in touch with this cycle is simple. Just use *Insight into Peace 1*. Knowing that you have no real physical hunger tells you that something else is going on. If you do *Insight into Peace 1* every time you *think* you have real physical hunger then you will soon realise there is a pattern to your behaviour. A good way to identify the pattern is to record your observations in your journal. What time of day did you have no real physical hunger—but wanted to eat anyway? Did you eat? What was it? How did you feel afterward? Make as many observations as you can about what you ate and how you felt at the time.

Once you see the pattern you will realise that it is not about the food. There are things in your life causing you pain. They may be big issues such as a traumatic childhood patterns or being caught in an unhappy relationship. At first, though, you will probably notice the smaller things. I used to eat after I had an argument with one of the kids, if I didn't get my own way or if I had spoken up at a staff meeting. When my emotions became too strong to deal with, eating or thinking about my diet were the only options for me.

There was nothing special that happened in my life that enabled me to make the decision to stop the diet and binge cycle. It came down to a simple question.

Do I wish to remain obsessed with food thoughts or do I want to live another way? I had to ask myself this question several times. Each time I would move forward a little more on the journey. My ultimate goal was not to lose weight. This is very important. **Losing weight is a by-product of finding peace with who you are.** So there is no real destination or goal on this journey. You are continually reassessing where you are, how you got here and how to move on without obsessing about food.

How do I manage this? I think in a completely different way than I did before. I stay in the moment as much as possible. Staying in the moment allows me to connect with life rather than with food. When my thoughts do wander to food and I have no real physical hunger I ask myself "What is this food story about?" I acknowledge my feelings. I connect with other things besides food like going for a morning walk, feeling myself smile or watching my son do his skateboarding tricks. This helps me to stay in the now, and helps me appreciate what I have.

Before I get out of bed every morning I visualise the day ahead and focus on the positive. I focus on the interactions I expect to have with people. I imagine how they will respond to me, how they will smile. I get in touch with how my body feels.

I am grateful for all the energy I will bring to this day, and for all the energy this day will bring to me. When you wake tomorrow morning try this: before you open your eyes listen to the sounds around you. What can you hear? Birds? The wind? The trees rustling in the breeze? Connect with nature. If you hear the kids or other noise, tune out, and listen for the sounds of nature. If you find this difficult, get a relaxation CD to play in the morning. Connect with these beautiful sounds. Ask yourself what you are grateful for today. It may be as simple as waking up to these sounds! You may have a deity you wish to thank for what you will receive today. Imagine that your day will run perfectly. Consider each detail in your mind. If you start to feel stressed, then slow down. Visualise a new approach for the cranky boss or a novel way to deal with a tight deadline. The thoughts you have right now will set the scene for the entire day. Make them count.

Time for Action

Once you have made your decision you will receive a call to action. The action reinforces your decision. It enables you to bring your decision to fruition on a day-to-day basis. When you take the action you commit to your decision, and it becomes a self-fulfilling prophecy. Once you decide to end your dieting and your food obsession, you will begin to focus on what is really eating you. This will give you the impetus you need to move towards peaceful eating.

The secret is simple: act as if you already have what you want.

This is how you turn a decision into a self-fulfilling prophecy. Imagine the things that you want in your life as though they have already happened. By doing this you focus on the positive, rather than the negative. You give your energy to what you want instead of what you don't want.

Make this moment your time for action. Start with the easiest step: consider the food you eat. Have plenty of food you love available. Analyse any food that you wish to eat based on *Insight into Peace 2*. Don't compromise on taste. If it is not the best, then choose something else. Go shopping. Buy the food you love. Then eat it. Eating food you love shows love for yourself. You are telling yourself that you are worth it.

Don't settle for second best because that will lead you to eat food that you don't really want. Imagine having exactly what you want when you want it. You will feel satisfied physically and emotionally. You will have honoured yourself and your body by eating what you love.

I have chosen to eat organic food wherever possible. I used to wonder what all the fuss was about and thought that an apple was an apple, whether it was organic or not. Apples always seemed like such a chore to eat and were definitely a "diet food." They didn't seem to have much taste or were soft and floury. I only ate them to fill the gap between two main meals during a strict diet regimen. In fact, dieting was my main reason for eating most fruit and vegetables. They seemed to be bland, boring and tasteless. No wonder I avoided buying fruit and vegetables for so long. They were reserved as diet food.

Now I find so much joy in eating organic fruit and vegetables. The first time I ate an organic strawberry I realised that was how strawberries are supposed to taste. Having only ever eaten supermarket fruit and vegetables, I suddenly understood why strawberry jam was invented! Organic fruit is so much sweeter that I find I eat less because I am satisfied sooner. As I found peace with food, my body craved the natural sweetness of fruit over sugary foods such as lollies and biscuits. So whenever possible I always choose organic food over other food.

By supporting cafes and restaurants that choose organic produce you are saying you want the best quality food. By supporting these businesses you are making peace with yourself. You are honouring the use of local, fresh, minimally processed, pesticide and chemical free food. It is good for you and it is good for the environment.

Decisions about food go hand-in-hand with decisions about exercise. These decisions are important. You choose to exercise because you feel good and healthy. Exercise makes you vibrant. Your body is designed to move, and the more you exercise, the better you understand your body. My favourite exercise is walking. I use my walking time as thinking time. I have made the decision to walk each day. (See *Insight into Peace 28.*) Find your dream exercise. If you haven't exercised for some time, look for a beginners' class in yoga or take the dog for a walk. Allocate time in your diary and commit to following through.

Exercise will come naturally when you realise that it is an expression of self-love. You will want to move. I was surprised to find that I often jog during my walk. My body naturally wants to go faster. I know when enough is enough but I actually enjoy the challenge of moving quickly. My body craves the healthy attention and if I miss a day it is not the same. Imagine yourself being open to the exercise that is right for you. Close your eyes and imagine your heart beating faster, your breath nourishing the cells of your body as it takes in increased oxygen.

Where are you? Are you inside or outside? Can you get in touch with your surroundings? What are you doing? Are you walking, running, playing a team sport, or something else? How do you feel? Energised, happy, mentally alert? Now is the time to make it happen. Use what you have written to select the exercise that feels right for you.

So where do you start? Start now by eating food you love and exercising with passion. The very next time you feel real physical hunger, eat the food you love. Use the hunger scale (see *Insight into Peace 1*) to measure this. At first you may not be sure whether you have real physical hunger or not. Listen to your body. If you are unsure, wait fifteen minutes, and then check again. The more you learn to read your real physical hunger the better you will understand what is really going on. When there is no real physical hunger but you want to eat notice the feeling. Where is it? Can you relate its position to the chakras? How does it feel? Give it a name so that you may address it. Each time you do this you will become more familiar with the feelings you have. These feelings are normal!

At first, you may experience some emotional emptiness. After all, you have been covering this emptiness with food or food thoughts for too long. It is okay to feel this emptiness and recognise that you want to fill it. This emptiness is the key to your food obsession. Be curious about it without judging or criticising yourself. Take time to consider what it is all about. See what feelings emerge. Do food thoughts take over again? Where do your thoughts take you when you go beyond thinking about food? Do you want to follow those thoughts? What are your choices? Do you want to continue the food obsession or do you want to find your peace?

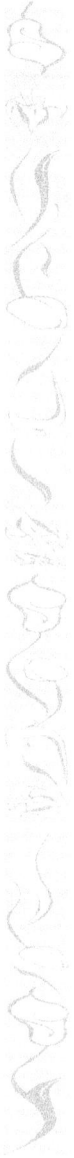

5

Find Your Peace

CLOSE YOUR EYES AND IMAGINE "PEACE." What do you see, hear or feel? Can you feel anything or is your life too chaotic to even contemplate peace? Does peace seem like a distant goal? To have peace in our lives we need to know and understand what peace is.

Does Anyone Know What Peace is Anyway?

If you have never experienced peace, how do you know what it is? Peace means different things to different people, but there are common elements. I asked some people for their thoughts about peace. Some of their responses were:

Any time I can get quiet, watch my breath, move into stillness, the peace is always there,

waiting for me to show up.
                    —Meera, Glenn, United States

Inner peace is within. Sometimes I need to shift my vision from what seems immediate to feel its presence again. It's just a shift of perspective.
                    —Jane Teresa, Brisbane, Australia

I find peace daily whenever decisions are made from my spirit and going with my natural feelings first and foremost. Whenever I tend to fight this and put too much logic into the equation, peace is always lost. Trusting myself is where the peace is found. Peace can occur regardless of external circumstances. It is never sourced externally by things or others. It can occur amidst great upset and sadness just as it can through joy, laughter and fun. Its source comes from within, just like happiness, but you must trust yourself to discover it.
                    —Nicole, Gold Coast, Australia

Inner peace is our natural state.
                    —Jim, California, United States

Inner peace is a state where you are free of negative thoughts, and feel a warm, golden, inner glow. It is being completely comfortable with who you are and not wishing you were any different, physically or emotionally. It is being able to deal with anything life throws at you and just get on with 'being'.

—Caro, Brisbane, Australia

These statements show us that peace comes from within. It emerges from our inner core. We cannot find peace in the world outside. Money, relationships, food—none of these can bring us peace. To find peace, we need to look within. Whenever I speak of "within", I speak of my inner core.

This may be scary to those of us who have avoided looking inside. We use food to save ourselves from introspection. We don't have to think about our inner core when food demands all our attention. Our obsession with food keeps us in our heads, thinking and problem solving, criticising and judging. Our obsession with food keeps us from finding our true peace.

When we find the peace that comes from within, it frees us from judgement and self-criticism. We experience compassion—compassion for others, and compassion for ourselves. We allow things to happen. We have no reason to hide from our inner core.

My inner core is like a bright candle. It used to be flickering in the wind, a whisper away from being extinguished. Now when I visualise my inner core, it burns brightly, lighting the way for me to see where I need to go and what I need to do. It keeps me going. You may have a name you wish to use for your inner core. If you give your inner core its own personal name it will help you to connect with it. It will be familiar to you and you will get to know it even better if you give it a name that you feel comfortable with.

It is important to identify how your inner core feels to you, so you will know where to find the peace within. To do this take a moment to close your eyes and breathe, noticing each breath as you inhale and exhale. Scan your entire body. Start at your head and work your way down your body, noticing the sensations you feel within. Look for the centre. Where is your soul? Your heart? Your inner being? With each breath focus closer on this area. What does it look like? Is it a shape, colour or symbol? Does it feel strong or weak, or does it flicker in intensity? Ask for a name. What does it say? This is your inner core talking to you. At any time you choose, you can go back to this moment to experience your inner core. Use this technique when you need to connect with yourself.

This is how you create your peace. Imagine each time you feel your emotions coming up that you are able to connect with your inner core. Visualise and feel the effects of those emotions on your spirit. Your inner core will connect you with the universe. You and the universe are one. Remember that the process of losing weight involves your body, mind and spirit. While you are connecting with your inner core is a good time to explore the power of your chakras. In Chapter Two I introduced each of the chakras—the root, sacral, solar plexus, heart, throat, third eye and crown chakras. Coming to peace with the spirit means that all your chakras are in balance. Your chakras are your inner energy. Once the chakras are in balance your energy becomes lighter, and flows more easily.

Take a moment to visualise your chakras. You can do this by focussing on each chakra point on your body and imagining the corresponding coloured light.

Root	*Red*
Sacral	*Orange*
Solar Plexus	*Yellow*
Heart	*Green*
Throat	*Blue*
Third Eye	*Indigo*
Crown	*Purple*

Measure the intensity of the light. Is it strong and pulsating, or dull and weak? Chakras open and close according to our emotions, so if the colour is dull and weak this may indicate that some emotions are interfering with your natural peaceful state. The position of the chakra may give an indication of the emotion. For example, if your heart chakra is weak, what matters of the heart are affecting you right now? Relationship issues? Family? Or if you feel your throat chakra is weak, what do you feel you are prevented from saying? Are there any communication issues affecting you right now? When we are at peace each chakra emanates pulsating light. Use the chakras as a guide to what may be happening in your life right now. If you discover an issue, imagine that the light is intense and bright. This may also allow a feeling to surface—a feeling that tells you what you need to do to clear the blockage.

Surrender

Letting go of our food obsession is the key to finding peace with ourselves. Letting go means surrendering our obsessions. When we surrender, we allow ourselves to experience our feelings and move through them. There is a knowing that allows me to surrender to this experience without fear. I know that I will come out the other side without the world crashing down on me. The worst thing that can happen to me is that I will *feel* my feelings. It will be the same for you.

By not eating unless we are physically hungry, we allow ourselves space. When we are not used to this space, it can feel very uncomfortable. Surrender to this uncomfortable feeling. It's the only way to move beyond the discomfort. In the past, we filled this space with food, rather than dealing with our uncomfortable feelings.

Here is the process I use when I surrender to these feelings. I let go. In the place of those uncomfortable feelings, I give myself over to a feeling of emotional fullness. I focus on my inner core. I breathe into it and give it life. I imagine my flame burning strongly. I feel the feelings that go with this in mind, body and spirit. My inner core comes alive. I have surrendered to the feeling of life. This brings me peace. My inner core grows stronger every time I surrender to my feelings.

By now you should understand there is no control in this approach to peaceful eating. The difference between control and surrender is that when I am in control I am at war with food. Control still means obsession with food. It doesn't allow me to acknowledge my feelings. Control is regimented and rule-bound. When something goes wrong all hell breaks loose. Trying to control your food intake distracts you from those aspects of life that you can't control. It is an illusion. Your emotions will still be there long after the food is gone, and long after you have begun your next diet. Control gives you a false sense of security and tricks your mind into thinking that "Everything will be okay once I lose the weight." You can avoid dealing with your feelings now and save them for later—once you have lost weight.

The problem is that this never happens. You will never feel good enough, and there is always another diet or binge around the corner to solve all your problems.

If you feel like you want to take control, take a breath instead. Focus on your inner core and allow your light to shine. It is time to surrender and work with peace. Surrender means giving up your old diets and food obsessions. Surrender means finding your peace.

Make Peace with the Past

Another way to ensure that your peace is fully present is to make peace with the past. For me, the same feelings from childhood kept coming up over and over again. They seemed to emerge in different forms but their essence was always the same. Emotional clearing is a very powerful technique. I had the good fortune to participate in two emotional clearing workshops. During these workshops I was able to connect with my childhood trauma and found the missing part of the puzzle. I was missing my mother's arms! I needed the protection and love of her hugs—hugs which I so rarely received. Instead, I had comforted myself with food. Only through those workshops could I recognise and truly connect with my need for my mother's hugs. Sadly, she passed away many years ago, so I had to find my peace with her some other way. By visualising the love and protection I had always wanted from my mother, I shifted something in my heart. I created a positive, loving experience without resorting to food, and this brought me peace with the past.

If you feel that you need professional guidance with this process, please contact a practitioner experienced in emotional clearing. If you are ready to look deeply into your past, you can begin your own emotional clearing.

To do this, think of your issue with food. How long has food had a negative impact on your life? What thoughts, words and images come to your mind? Connect with the feelings of your war on food.

Focus on the chakras that you find are most weak. Next, think of an image from childhood that stirs up negative emotions. It doesn't have to be related to the first image of food; whatever comes into your mind first is the image to work with. How did you see the world as a child? Did you feel unsafe? Scared? Untrusting? Helpless? Hopeless? Make a list of all the emotions that you felt. Next, write down how you coped with those emotions. Did you eat? Starve? Withdraw? Become angry? Or did you do something else? The next step requires you to make a choice. Do you want to choose peace with this issue? If your answer is "Yes", affirm it with the words "I choose peace." If the answer is "No", ask yourself why you have made this choice. What needs are you fulfilling by continuing to hold onto this issue? If I choose to hold onto a negative emotion or stance such as withdrawal, this may keep me from committing to a job or a relationship. This means that you may need some imagined security, at the expense of happiness, love, or exploring the world.

Your emotional needs may keep you trapped in some negative core beliefs about yourself. Believing that you are hopeless stops you from moving forward in life. It is a good excuse if you plan to stay in a relationship that isn't working, or a job that is destroying your soul. But just imagine that you don't need to feel hopeless anymore. How would your life change? It would change everything. This may sound too difficult to even attempt. But you don't have to attempt anything. All you have to do is affirm peace.

Once you affirm your desire to choose peace, visualise your childhood image again. What do you feel you want to add or remove from the image? How can you make this image peaceful? For me, it was as simple as visualising my mother's arms wrapped around me, protecting me during my most vivid childhood traumas, such as those times when the boys continually tormented me. There may be emotions that you release during this visualisation. Continue your affirmation while the emotions are released. This is a good time to use essential oil support (see *Appendix*). Using your journal to write about your feelings will also help.

War ... What is it Good For?

In the absence of war, it seems logical that there is peace. After the war, we come to peace. We have already discovered that there is more to peace than simply deciding that our war with food is over. When we decide not to participate in the war, we change our mindset—and we take action. If we refuse to change our behaviour, how can we say the war has ended?

We need to take positive steps towards our peace. We need to change our relationship with food. Food is no longer our enemy; after the war, it must become our friend. This can be challenging, because we have used food to cover up our pain, hurt and other negative feelings. Making peace in other areas of our lives seems to follow naturally once we make our peace with food. This way, we begin to acknowledge the changes that we need to make.

When the battle is over the bombing stops and everything falls quiet. But it doesn't end there. Keeping our distance seems the first step, then it is time to negotiate with our inner core. We finally listen to both sides, including our heart, rather than listening to our negativity. The negotiation keeps us moving towards agreement, resolution, and the future. You have made some decisions and performed some actions to support your food choices.

You have also identified that the past plays a significant part in finding peace. Now you also need to deal with the future. War plays no part in your future. You are looking forward to what can be, rather than looking back at what has passed. Focussing on the future rather than dwelling in the past will propel you in the direction you need to go. War is good for absolutely nothing.

Be a Peace Activist

To create peace around food we need to take action in other aspects of our lives. The outspoken American journalist Dorothy Thompson (1894-1961) was quoted as saying, "Peace has to be created, in order to be maintained. It is the product of Faith, Strength, Energy, Will, Sympathy, Justice, Imagination, and the triumph of principle. It will never be achieved by passivity and quietism." The same principle applies when we believe that our personal war with food is over, and we act on our beliefs. To create peace we first focus on food as fuel. We then focus on the feelings we have and how we deal with them.

If we think that peace will "just happen", we are kidding ourselves. We have to look for peace, understand it, value it and then use it as our underlying philosophy about who we are.

I used to eat but I still felt empty. I didn't know why that was. I did know that if I continued eating I would never stop and this was my signal that something was not quite right. Now I understand that my emptiness was the raw emotion that I had never previously allowed myself to feel. Now I embrace the feeling. Here is how you can work towards embracing your emotions rather than forcing them down with food:

When you feel you want to eat ask yourself, "Is it real physical hunger?" If it is, follow the approach for choosing the most peaceful food for you at this time. If not, it is time to embrace this lesson. Ask yourself, "What is my body trying to teach me?" Take a breath and be still for a moment. Notice the area of your body which feels uncomfortable. Give it a name—is it your inner core or soul talking? Is it a particular emotion talking? Listen to it. What does it want to tell you? If it could speak what would it say? Ask it what you need right now. You can choose to eat if you make it purposeful, or you can choose not to eat. Complete a relevant *Insight into Peace*. For example, if you choose to eat, *Insight into Peace 16—Eating to Cover Emotions* may be relevant. If you want to deal with feelings choose *Insight into Peace 13—Real Pain*.

By learning how to embrace your feelings when you have no real physical hunger, you will be able to work out what is really eating you.

Peace is Fun

My friend and I were talking about what peace meant to her. After some discussion she said, "Mundane life necessities are not peaceful." Before I could comment she added something else: "Or maybe they could be, and that's where I'm going wrong?" I felt that she was right on the mark. If you are struggling with everything around you—what to cook for dinner or the challenges of your working life—then do something about these problems. Take action. Peace should be fun in all aspects of your life. If peace is not fun, it means that you have not discovered the true feeling of peace. Imagine these two scenarios. You get home from work, too tired to cook. You look in the freezer. There is a packet of frozen vegetables and a couple of chops to cook. You microwave the vegetables, fry the chops, and voila! Dinner is on the table. The second scenario begins the same way. You arrive home from work, tired but looking forward to a fresh salad. You chop the baby spinach, tomatoes, feta and olives, toss in some protein and drizzle with balsamic vinegar. Your food is alive so you also feel alive. Think about those frozen vegetables. Can you truly say that they still possess their life force?

Decide that you will perform your next task with peace in mind. This will mean connecting with your inner core, and allowing yourself to perform peacefully. Just as I choose peaceful food, I also choose peaceful household products. I only use chemical free cleaning or personal products. This way, I am continually affirming that I support peace in every aspect of my life. Being aware of the environment, the companies you are supporting and the packaging they use brings everyday peace. See the true value in everything that you do, whether it is a mundane task or a special event. Connect with your inner core and see beyond those things that you have covered up for so long.

When you find your peace you will find that everything starts to take on a new perspective. Food is no longer a major focus of your life. You can deal peacefully with your feelings. Peace becomes an active part of your life. Now it is time to live your dream. Let's explore ways to bring your dream to life.

6

Bring Your Dream to Life

ARE YOU HAPPY? This is a simple question that requires a simple answer. If your answer is "No," then what is stopping you from bringing your dream to life? When I first met my partner he used to ask me, "Are you happy?" I never answered him. I was so scared of my gut reaction: "No." It wasn't about him. It was about how I reacted to life. I felt insecure in our relationship, asking myself how I could deserve such a nice guy who treated me well. I was so used to being treated badly. It seemed he loved me for who I was! Just as my understanding of myself has changed, so has my understanding of our relationship. My partner and I have a relationship that is both equal and caring. I have learned to love myself as he loves me. Now when he asks me if I am happy, my answer is "Yes." And guess what? It is no coincidence that I now eat peacefully too.

The steps which brought me to this place of peace are simple. I decided to end my war with food. I actively engaged in practices to find my peace. As a result, I discovered my dream. My dream is to participate fully in life. It sounds so simple but it took me a long time to get here. Earlier, I called this "walking the bridge." It is time to get over the bridge of your self-doubt and stop making excuses. As you discovered in the previous chapter, peace is not passive. Peace demands action. Bringing your dream to life demands action, too.

To live a life you must do something. If you didn't do anything you would die. What can you do today to make difference to your life? When food is not your focus, you need to find something to fill the space. This space is where our real issues reside. It is when we feel uncomfortable with this space that food thoughts come to mind.

What Do You Really Want?

Try this for a few minutes. Put down the book and just sit. Observe your own mind. Don't get caught up in any thoughts. When you find yourself thinking, say to yourself, "There you are thinking about (whatever it is) again." Let those thoughts float away on a cloud. Each time a thought enters let it float away on a cloud. There is no need to make anything happen. Just allow the cloud to take the thought away.

When you feel that you have cleared you mind it is time to dream. Imagine you have everything you always wanted and the goals that you have written down previously in Chapter 4 are all coming true. You are living the life you want without resistance. Ask yourself, "What is the very next thing I need to do?" Let your answer come as a feeling or image. This works best if you don't indulge in problem solving or critical thinking. Allow your answer to come from your inner core. Your answer will lead you in the right direction. You might allow yourself more time to yourself, or you may spend more time studying your favourite hobby. You may even write the outline for your first book!

Focussing on the next step gives us a new mini-goal each time we look at the big picture.

Feeling Connected

So what is different? The difference is that each day I feel committed and connected. You may be wondering what it means to "be connected"? It means being connected to something other than food and dieting. In my case, being connected has given me the freedom to do whatever I wish, without the fear of the food war. It comes down to three simple steps:

- ❧ Awareness
- ❧ Allowing
- ❧ Action

Awareness

Begin this step by focussing your attention on some key questions. Who am I? Where am I in my life? What is my place in the world? Previously, you have written down some goals about relationships, career, family and self. Now it is time to do something with those goals. Writing the goals is an important step, but what you do next is just as important. You have to bring your consciousness to the next step. This is awareness. Each morning I know my life has changed. I wake up with new thoughts and great ideas. I constantly have awareness that I am different.

This is a time to focus on your inner core (or the name you have given it) and breathe in your awareness. Doing this at the beginning of each morning is a great way to envisage how you want the day to unfold. In previous chapters, I have explored different ways to greet the day with gratitude. You are welcome to expand upon these ideas. Ask yourself, "What will be different today?" Challenge yourself to make positive changes: "If there was one thing that I could change about today, it would be ..."

Once again, your answer will come spontaneously. Perhaps it will be an image, or a feeling. Make a commitment to follow through with your answer. During the day, bring your awareness back to your answer often. When you notice that you are following through, give yourself the gratitude you deserve.

You will become aware of the vibrational frequency you are emitting. Frequency is a subtle form of energy. Other people pick up on your frequency. For example, imagine you wake up in the morning and it feels like nothing can go right. You get in the car and it refuses to start. When you get to work you find a pile of work on your desk. You miss an important phone call and then spill coffee all over your paperwork. You just knew the day was going to be terrible! You might not know it, but you are emitting a negative frequency.

Now compare your day to mine. Imagine that we work in the same office. I woke up with a wonderful intention that today would bring me one step closer to my goal. I smile at the boss and my team mates, and they all smile back. Others offer to help me with some paperwork, and the important proposal I had put forward has just been approved. I have chosen to emit a positive frequency. If I see you in the lunch room later in the day, I will pick up on your low frequency. Please don't take it personally, but I'll probably do my best to avoid you. The energy that you are emitting tends to drive people away. This is the difference between having a good day and a bad day.

Affirming your intention for the day gives awareness to what is possible. Success builds upon success. Positive energy supports more positive energy. When you start to feel a shift in your energy, everything will become much clearer. As your awareness develops you will be able to take more positive actions.

Action

We have already discussed in a previous chapter how the actions you take demonstrate the level of peace in your life. Now you are going to take it one step further by embracing the life you deserve. The best way to embrace the life you deserve is to act as if you already have everything you could want. Act as if you are living your dream; act as if you have it all. How would your life be different? How would you be different? What about your expectations of yourself and others? How would you expect others to treat you? Don't wait until you get to the "perfect" weight. Perfectionism sets us up for failure. We can have it all and we can have it all now. Write down all those things that you wanted to do when you lost weight. One of my dreams was to go to Europe. I wanted to go there once I had lost weight, once I felt that I was perfect in every way. Last year I made a decision. I chose to book the trip because I wanted an experience of a lifetime. I didn't wait for that perfect time that never comes. I acted as if I deserved to live my dreams. My trip to Europe was my fortieth birthday present to myself.

Once you have made your list, decide when you will do the items on your list. Do not base this decision on the amount of weight you will lose. Base it on your own timeline, and act as if it is part of your life now.

The same thing goes for the quality of food and resources you choose. To continue to live a peaceful life, choose peaceful foods that support local farmers and their families where possible. Fresh organic food tastes good, and is good for the environment as well. Packaged and processed foods do not bring peace; instead, they bring chaos. By consciously making a decision about the quality of food you eat you are taking action. You are saying that you are good enough and deserve the best at all times. You are responsible for your own actions.

Allowing

Do you try to take control of every situation that you encounter? When you are used to controlling your diet and your food cravings, it is inevitable that you will also try to control other parts of your life. When you try to control everything so tightly, cracks are bound to appear. As you know, this is when we turn to food to control all those unruly emotions. But there is another alternative.

One of the most amazing techniques I have ever learned is *allowing*. This means accepting that we have no control over anything. We can't make anyone do anything. And the more we try to control our own actions, the more we set impossible goals for ourselves.

This was a difficult thing for me to internalise as I was so used to perfectionism. When I didn't achieve perfection I beat myself up even further by eating more or following a more restrictive diet. This led me to focus on the food, rather than focussing on the real issue.

When I learned to allow things to take their natural course, I learned how I could have it all.

Make no mistake: allowing is not the same as doing nothing. Allowing means trusting the actions you take. Instead of control, the secret is to trust. Trust in yourself, and in your own judgement.

You may want to experiment with this. Start with any food issue. You may examine your hunger and discover that you are not physically hungry at all. You have a hunger that you don't understand. Trust that the answer will come. You may or may not recognise the reasons why you feel this hunger, but you may be curious about them, even though they cannot be explained physically. You will learn to allow these reasons and answers to come, rather than beating yourself up.

You have already discovered the power of your curiosity. Being curious and open-minded is a good way to examine what else might be going on. The second part of this process is to allow insight to develop by trusting your intuition and feelings. When you think about your food issue, does a word or a feeling pop into your mind? Do you get an image?

This is your intuition working to show you what is really eating you. When you allow this to develop you will find that each time you discover you are not physically hungry you will get a deeper insight into the issue. You will then be able to deal with it and allow the dreams you wish for to take the place of your hunger.

Life Brings Issues

Sometimes we have things we need to deal with on a day-to-day basis. Some of those are food issues and some are life issues. When we bring our dream to life, we find that it is better to learn than to judge. We are kind to ourselves and want the best for ourselves. Imagine you were your own best friend. How do you treat your best friends? Do you judge their actions or do you support them? Do you tell them everything they are doing wrong and chastise them? There is a saying that you must love yourself before you can love others. The things that you don't like in other people are usually a reflection of yourself.

Even something as simple as having a cup of tea with a friend can be a challenge some days. I have to be my own best friend first. One day I met a friend for morning tea. I decided not to have my usual cup of tea at breakfast, knowing I would have one with my friend. When I arrived at her place I found her making a hot white chocolate for the both of us. She was hand beating the milk on the stove and frothing it to perfection. She had also baked a fruit slice, and looked like she had gone to a lot of trouble. One problem: I definitely wasn't physically hungry. For a fleeting second I thought about saying "No thank you, I have just eaten." But I didn't. I let my friend serve me the beautifully made food and drink and I knew the moment I took my first sip that I was not going to make peace with this food.

As I ate and drank I became very aware of my stomach filling and bloating. Not long after that I noticed that my attention span was limited. Concentrating on what my friend was saying took a real effort.

When I returned home I felt very guilty about the food I had just eaten. I started to look for more food. Then I stopped, and I asked myself what I really wanted. I used some essential oils and wrote in my journal. I discovered some important issues I hadn't addressed.

What would have happened if I honoured myself and had a cuppa at my friend's house instead of accepting food and drink that did not agree with me? Would my day have been any different?

And why didn't I say "No thank you" to my friend. I didn't want to hurt her feelings! I was worried how she might react if I didn't eat her slice, and drink her hot chocolate. So what does that say about me? I don't like confrontation, I like to please, and it seemed easier than trying to say "No." What did that do for me? Absolutely nothing! I would have loved to take a slice home instead of eating it, but I didn't or wouldn't ask. I wanted to be a good friend and acknowledge the trouble she had gone to. In actual fact I could have easily been a good friend, while also looking after my own needs. There was nothing stopping me from telling her how much I appreciated the effort she had made, but that I would prefer to eat something plainer. I just didn't acknowledge my own needs at the time.

So what could I do about it? Nothing! I could only look at the episode honestly, without judgement on my part. The day was done. I couldn't go back. All I would do was change the way I responded next time. I learned from this lesson. What I learned is that I MUST acknowledge my needs, while also being appreciative of the person who is offering her hospitality.

Since that incident my friend and I have discussed my feelings about that day. At that time it was the beginning of our friendship so we had not discussed food in any detail. When the topic came up my friend said, "I should have asked you if the food and drink were suitable for you." That also taught me a lesson—to understand that everything is not my fault! I realised that my friend did not know me well enough to know my food needs—but nor did she take the time to ask.

Sometimes events will trigger memories of the past, leading us back to old habits. My dad visited me unannounced recently. He knew what to say to get my feelings flowing to the surface. "Have you put on weight?" I regressed immediately. I was the hurt little girl again.

I headed straight to the refrigerator, looking for something to fill the void inside. As I walked towards the kitchen I recognised the feeling. I went back and worked through the outline in *Insight into Peace 1*. When I assessed myself against the hunger scale, I realised that I was not physically hungry. Other emotions were being stirred up. The old feeling of hopelessness was coming to the surface. When you feel this emotional turmoil, it is important to understand what is happening. I had to deal with my feelings. Using *Insight into Peace 11* enabled me to connect with my inner child. She felt judged and criticised. I was able to tell my father how his words had hurt me. It was interesting to note that he didn't stay very long after this discussion.

When we face our ups and downs we have a choice: we can deal with them, or we can avoid them. We can accept the false comfort that food offers us, or we can face our fears and dreams. I believe that our fears and dreams are like yin and yang. They are interconnected. Fears hold us back from our dreams, but only when we confront our fears do we achieve our dreams. Believing in ourselves and trusting our feelings are essential if we are to trust in who we are. Once we trust our feelings we can leave our food and diet obsession behind.

It is Not the Destination it is The Journey

By now you will probably realise that losing weight peacefully is never going to be a quick fix. Peacefulness takes work and the path to peace takes work. It means making decisions on a daily basis about what is best for you. Losing weight is a by-product of this journey.

Sometimes you will look back to see how far you have come. Looking back is okay. I also felt some grief when I lost the old me, because I had relied on her for so long. It is like losing a friend who you know is not good for you. You know you have to move on because the friendship is destroying you. Your friend is sucking the life out of you, but you can't help being attracted to her in some strange way. If you have ever experienced such a demanding friendship, you will know that once you made the break you became so much happier. You wonder why you didn't do it earlier; you wonder why you wasted so much time and energy with that person. The reason is that you had a lesson you needed to learn. And once you had learned it, you were ready to move on. When you look back your insight is clear. You know why you made the break, but sometimes you feel a pang of regret. Still, you are wise enough to know that it could not have ended any other way.

You know that you must lead your life without your old friend.

Food and dieting can feel the same as a demanding friendship. You feel drawn to the next diet or binge, but when you look at it objectively, you see how destructive it would be. Dieting and binging will bring more pain, and you would only be using your food obsession to cover up some strong emotions. You know this obsession is not good for your soul, so it is time to leave diets and binging behind for good. You have many discoveries to make and your new vision will allow you to continue over the bridge to the new land. Having people in your life who support you with this is so important. Do you have people in your life you know that will support you and honour you? Or do you feel like they suck your energy with every breath you take? Release yourself from any energies that are holding you back. This may mean distancing yourself from a friend who is clingy, or a relationship that is based on put-downs.

I now know the real me. She is allowed to say what she wants, and allowed to be who she wants. Connecting with my needs at any given moment provides a basis for peaceful eating. I choose food that allows me to honour myself, food that is good for me and good for the environment. Changing my mindset has led me to peaceful living. When I choose peace I choose all the joy that comes with it. Right now I bring my dream to life, which means I can choose to lose weight peacefully without diets, without my old food obsession. You too can bring your dream to life just by choosing peace. This is the change you have been looking for!

Insights into Peace:
Daily Practices

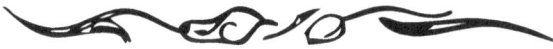

7

Food

FOOD WAS MY WAR. Now it is my peace. Each time I reach for food I make a choice about who I am. I can choose to be the person who uses food as an excuse, as something to stuff down and hide my emotions. Or I can use food as fuel—the way it was meant to be. When I am at peace with food, other aspects of my life seem to be manageable. When my life is chaotic, so are my food choices. Learning how to use food as fuel is a process of observation and selection. You can't do it unless you value yourself. When I don't value myself I will use whatever food it takes to influence my emotions and change the way I feel. When I do value myself I make rational food choices—choices I can believe in.

Starting with food choices is the beginning of change. The *Insight into Peace* practices allow you to examine your eating behaviour. You will start to appreciate and value food for the high quality fuel it will provide to your body. Each practice has a list of essential oils that have been matched for their emotional properties and their ability to support your feelings during the practice. To discover how to use the Essential Oil Support, see the *Appendix.*

You may follow the *Insight into Peace* practices in sequence. Alternatively, you can do one that catches your attention, or one that you feel is particularly relevant for you. Keep a record of your insights in your journal along with the date of the entry, so that you can look back on your progress towards losing weight peacefully.

Insight into Peace 1

Real Physical Hunger

My War: I ate when I was not physically hungry. I felt out of control and desperate. I didn't have balance in my life. Food filled the gap and evened out my emotions whether I was happy or sad, or when I didn't know how I felt. Food enabled me to numb myself and not think about the real issues.

My challenge was based on one question: What was the worst thing that could happen if I was to face the real issue? I could face it head on and have to deal with it. Or I could choose not to deal with it and eat anyway.

My Peace: The first step is to identify what *real physical hunger* is. For me, I start to feel light headed. I might even find a headache coming on. My stomach feels empty. Sometimes I get a little irritable, too. Then my stomach might start rumbling.

This is a gradual process. I can choose to finish what I am doing, then eat. I don't need to feel urgent about the need to eat.

I can monitor my physical hunger on a scale of one to ten. *One* being absolutely ravenous—this could be dangerous as I won't have the time to prepare something I really want. *Ten* is feeling absolutely stuffed to the point of being sick.

If I am *five* or above, it means I am not physically hungry.

To Do: Each time you want to eat, tune into your physical hunger. A good way to do this is to close your eyes and take a deep, slow breath in and out. Then ask yourself where the hunger is. Identify it in your body. Is your stomach rumbling? Does your stomach feel empty? Do you feel light headed or irritable? Is your hunger increasing gradually, or is it demanding immediate gratification? On a scale of one to ten, where are you now?

Eating when you are at *three* or *four* on the hunger scale is eating for real physical hunger. If you recognise that you are a *one* or *two*, be aware of the danger of over eating when you are ravenous.

You can choose to eat at any number. But now you are fully informed about your real physical hunger and you can make the wisest possible choice.

Essential Oil Support: Frankincense, Lavender, Sandalwood, Ylang Ylang.

Insight into Peace 2

Food I Love

My War: I thought about the food I really liked, compared it to the food I ate, and discovered they were not the same. Sometimes I made quick decisions or felt like I had to eat to fit in with what was being offered so I ate food I didn't really like. I realised when I love myself I made loving choices; when I didn't, I treated myself as second best.

My Peace: My plan is to make a list of foods I love. Not like, but **love**. Here is part of my list: strawberries, avocados, freshly brewed organic coffee, calamari, big green salad with balsamic vinegar, char-grilled red capsicum, Lindt chocolate … You get the idea.

So how do I know I love these foods? Because they make me feel good, both physically and emotionally. My soul sings. My heart doesn't feel like it is struggling under the pressure of greasy, over-processed food, my belly isn't bloated and I can breathe in with a full breath without feeling uncomfortable. I feel alive in a whole new way.

To Do: Make a list of food you love.

Use the following questions to determine if it is a food you love, like or dislike. Choose a food.

1. Look at the colour. What do you think of it? Natural? Artificial? Pretty? Bland?
2. Is the food local or imported? How far has it travelled?
3. Can you identify its raw ingredients by looking at it?
4. Are they quality ingredients? I am not talking about its calorie, carbohydrate or fat content. Are the ingredients natural, identifiable and real?
5. Smell the food. How does it smell? Sweet? Stale? Fresh? Ripe?
6. Look at the texture. Is it limp? Crisp and fresh? Fried? Grilled? Overcooked?
7. Take a bite. What is the first taste that comes to mind? Too sweet? Too salty? Too sour? Just right?
8. How do you feel after eating the food? Does it give you indigestion? Or do you feel crisp and clean? Energised? Comforted? Or tired? Heavy? Light?

Use as many senses as possible to identify if the food is *really a food you love.* You do not want to waste any more time on cheap and nasty food. You want value and satisfaction with each bite.

Make it count ... and I don't mean calories! Feel good about the food you eat because you love it.

Essential Oil Support: Lemon, Peppermint, Spearmint, Clary Sage.

Insight into Peace 3

The Next Meal

My War: When binging takes hold I don't know when to stop. The war can last for hours. But at some stage I will stop binging, and then I will be confronted by my next meal. The next meal scares me—I don't want to start binging again.

My Peace: I am in touch with my feelings and I understand there is a reason for my binging, whether before, during or after the episode. The reasons may be clear to me at the beginning and I choose to eat anyway. I discover these reasons, learn from them, and decide I want peace in my life.

To Do: No matter how long it is since you have binged, make the commitment that you will eat the very next time you have real physical hunger. Continue to check in with yourself and rate your hunger using the hunger scale.

Essential Oil Support: Black Pepper, Frankincense, Cedarwood, Cinnamon.

Insight into Peace 4

Serving Size

My War: I used to pile my plate high with vegetables or salads. I thought I was doing myself a favour by eating huge amounts of food that was good for me. But I still believed that I had to stuff myself until I was full.

My Peace: Having an average size meal satisfies my real physical hunger. It does not matter what the food is as long as it is a food I love. When I started going to the local organic cafe, I noticed the size of the meals were smaller than I was used to but I felt completely satisfied.

To Do: Go to a second hand shop and find an old plate. In the 1960s serving sizes were much smaller. We were given a set and the diameter of the serving section of the plate was eighteen centimetres. I compared that to a modern set I own, and found that the diameter across the modern plate was twenty-three centimetres. That is a five centimetre increase in a couple of decades. Do you need the large plate? Consider that if you fill your plate, you have given yourself an extra five centimetres of food all round. Doesn't sound like much, does it? But if you fill a twenty-three centimetre plate, you have just given yourself a **60% *larger serving*** than that the eighteen centimetre plate. Is large normal? Make a decision that small is normal. You can always have seconds.

Go retro and match your appetite to your plate size!

Essential Oil Support: Patchouli, Benzoin, Vetiver, Cinnamon.

Insight into Peace 5

What to Eat

My War: Having lots of processed food in the house meant that I could easily fill up on cheap, low quality fuel any time. It was easy to eat chips or have a block of chocolate instead of the food my body actually wanted.

My Peace: I imagine that high quality, organic food has a soul. It has been made with love and care. Compared with conventional farming practices, its impact on the environment has been greatly reduced. No pesticides or chemicals have been used. There is no chemical warfare.

To Do: You may have already made a list of food you love. Now when you have real physical hunger, how do you decide what you want to eat? Spending some time with your senses will help you assess what your body really needs. Use your senses— sight, feel, taste and touch—to help decide what your body needs right now. Start with this list:

- ❧ Sweet or sour ?
- ❧ Spicy or salty?

- ❧ Smooth or crunchy?
- ❧ Hot or cold?
- ❧ Light or heavy?
- ❧ Soft or hard?
- ❧ A range of colours or one colour?

Here are some examples of how you can compare foods to find the one you really want: Is it the crispness of an apple or the softness of a strawberry? Does it feel light and cool like a salad or soft and warm like a casserole? Compare foods and see which one brings a spark to your feelings. You will feel the joy of preparing and eating the food. It will bring you pleasure.

Essential Oil Support: Bergamot, Lemon, Helichrysum, Jasmine.

Insight into Peace 6

Half-an-Hour Lunch Break

My War: I was in a stressful job. I didn't have a normal lunch break. I was expected to work through my lunch. Because I did, no one valued my time, including me. I always ate on the run. I bought junk food to fill up quickly, or ate at my desk. I never allowed myself the pleasure of enjoying food. I accepted that this was the way it was, and that I did not deserve to take time out for myself to refuel and recharge.

It also meant that I made up for it later in the day when I got home. I resented having to eat what I really didn't want to eat because I was rushed or stressed.

My Peace: Making the decision that I deserved to have a break to eat was one of the best decisions I ever made. I allowed myself the time and space to eat my food with peace. I chose an area where I could not be disturbed. If anyone interrupted me, I explained that I was on my lunch break, and I would be back in half-an-hour. At first this was hard to do, as it felt like I was being selfish. Others chose to work through their lunch breaks. Instead of eating quick filler foods that would leave me lethargic later in the afternoon, I believe I was more productive in the afternoon by allowing myself time to eat proper nourishing food.

To Do: Allow yourself to have **at least** a half-an-hour lunch break. Make the time. Cross off the half-hour in your diary. Do not sit at your desk. Find a comfortable place to sit, whether it is a lunch room, outside under a tree or in a cafe. You deserve to have a decent break. Take this as time to take in your nourishment for the afternoon. Learn to say, "I am on my lunch break; I'll see you in half an hour."

Essential Oil Support: Cedarwood, Coriander, Cypress, Ginger.

Insight into Peace 7

Impact of Food On Your Life

My War: Food was a constant struggle in my life. It stopped me from participating in life. I was too tired, too worn out or just too full from overeating! I wasted time, energy and money on diets and food obsession.

My Peace: Recognising that my diet and food obsession was there to hide my real feelings gives me a sense of relief. I started to understand that every time I ate when I wasn't physically hungry it was for a reason. Learning these reasons has allowed me to find peace with food.

To Do: Make a list of reasons that food has had a negative impact on your life. Make the number of reasons equal your age. For example: I am forty-one, so I would write forty-one reasons. While writing the list do it as quickly as you can without giving it too much thought. Compiling this list will allow your subconscious to give you some insight into the impact that food has had on your life.

You may choose to spend some time reflecting on your list and identifying any common elements.

Look for themes or repeated words. Once you see these write a summary about these themes. When you finish, observe your feelings around this summary. What is significant about the themes? Do they give you some insight into why you have chosen a food and diet obsession? Take some time to understand that when you eat peacefully you address these issues. Refer to your list regularly to gauge your progress.

Essential Oil Support: Pine, Melissa, Bay, Cypress.

Insight into Peace 8

Embrace the Quality

My War: I stuffed down my food and ate fast because I had not found my peace. I ate quickly so I wouldn't have to think about anything except how much I ate, how greedy I was or how bad I felt. I used food to numb any other emotion. I learnt not to feel. Food was my enemy, so I punished myself with it.

My Peace: Now I love the quality of the food that I provide for my family and myself. I can choose a food and truly believe that it is good for me and good for the planet—even if it is chocolate. I can enjoy my food, spend time with it and notice its unique feel, colours and tastes.

To Do: Examine your next meal. What colours and textures are on the plate? Taste each food separately. Identify each of the single ingredients. If you can't identify the single ingredients, ask yourself why not?

Which food do you *love*?

Which foods are just OK?

Which do you eat simply because they are in front of you?

Decide which foods have quality ingredients. Embrace quality food and make it count.

Essential Oil Support: Tangerine, Myrtle, Geranium, Ylang Ylang.

Insight into Peace 9

Organic

My War: My food displayed signs of war, too. Many of the foods I used to eat were processed, containing artificial flavours, colours and preservatives. The original ingredients were virtually unrecognisable. Even so-called "fresh" fruit and vegetables were bland, waxed and contained other additives to make them attractive for sale.

My Peace: Knowing the origins of my food brought a lightness that became part of my soul. My food tastes good and I know that I am supporting a sustainable world. Organic food is grown without pesticides and sold without additives. It is good for me, the farmer and the farmer's family. I know that I am eating quality food that has been ethically grown. This is peaceful food.

To Do: Do the organic taste test. Find your local reputable organic store. Buy your favourite fruit or vegetable and compare it with the same food purchased from a supermarket. Notice the appearance of the fruit or vegetable. Apples are a perfect example. An organic apple may have some marks, and seem to be a little on the small side. Supermarket apples are generally huge! They are waxed for a glossy appearance. Now take a bite! Which one tastes the way you expect an apple to taste? Supermarket apples usually taste bland. There is little difference in size, shape, colour or taste across the range. Compare this with the sweet juicy flavour of the organic apple. If you have been eating supermarket fruit and vegetables for some time you will definitely notice the amazing taste of organic produce. Enjoy!

If you live in a rural area look for online stores that are able to supply organic food, or grow your own. If you want to grow your own start with herbs, pumpkins and cherry tomatoes. These are low maintenance. Our pumpkins and tomatoes simply grew out of our compost!

Essential Oil Support: Basil, Oregano, Lemon, Orange.

Insight into Peace 10

Slow Down

My War: I ate so quickly that I did not taste the food on my plate. When I ate fast it was a sign that I was in my war with food. I was like an addict getting her fix. I had to scoff the food down fast to numb or suppress or divert my feelings. I didn't need to taste the food. I only needed it to cover up my emotions.

My Peace: When I eat slowly I take the time to appreciate my food. I use all my senses to relish the full experience of nourishing my body. I notice how my food smells, how it tastes, and how it feels in my mouth. I chew my food slowly. I am able to engage in social conversation rather than feeling distracted by the food. I am able to put my knife and fork down between bites and give myself the time to enjoy. I treat the food and my body with respect and reverence.

To Do: Take one sultana and observe it. Spend a few minutes thinking about where this sultana came from. Is it from a local organic source? Visualise the farmer, the vines, and the workers who harvest the fruit. Send them some gratitude for their work, which has brought this sultana to you today. What is its colour? Texture? Shape? Squish it a little. Is it plump and juicy or slightly dry and hard?

Put the sultana in your mouth and hold it between your teeth. What do you notice? Its sweetness, its hardness or softness, or something else? Move it into your mouth and allow your tongue to roll over it. Resist the temptation to bite! Notice how it feels and how your mouth responds. Slowly make your first bite and allow the sultana to sit a little longer in your mouth. Notice your body's reaction. Is there saliva building up? Is there an intense sweetness? Now chew the sultana slowly, taking a few minutes to allow it to move further around your mouth before you swallow. When you are ready, allow yourself to guide the sultana gently to the back of your mouth to be swallowed. Notice how your mouth and stomach feel now. You have just mindfully eaten a sultana.

Essential Oil Support: Ginger, Tangerine, Nutmeg, Cinnamon.

8

Feelings

*I*T WAS DIFFICULT FOR ME to express my real
feelings, especially when they were triggered
by pain from the past. Most of the time I was
unaware that some painful emotions had been
triggered. All I knew was that I was heading straight
for the fridge. I thought it was about the way someone
had just spoken to me or an argument I had just lost.
I could not see the patterns that had been occurring
in my life for a long time. All I knew was that I had
uncomfortable feelings and the best way to deal with
them was to eat. I had to learn to be curious about
my feelings. Then I had to learn new ways of dealing
with my feelings, instead of dieting or binging.

The *Insights into Peace* in this chapter allow you
to explore the relationship between food and your

feelings. Exploring this relationship will give you an awareness of what is really happening emotionally when you think of food. You will find out where the relationship between food and your feelings began. And you will learn how to distinguish between emotional hunger and real physical hunger. As you explore your feelings you will gain a deeper awareness of your emotional life. You will learn to deal with your feelings in a way that honours you.

Continue to use your journal to work through this chapter. Remember you may follow the *Insight into Peace* practices in sequence. Alternatively, you can do one that catches your attention, or one that you feel is particularly relevant for you. Spend as much time as you need to work through these practices, and revisit them as often as you like. The more you repeat these practices, the more you will gain.

Insight into Peace 11

What Are You Feeling?

My War: Sometimes I knew I was not physically hungry and I didn't know what I was really hungry for. To know this I have to identify the feelings that goes with my hunger. That is the hard part. I have avoided my feelings for so long, and I don't fully accept them for what they are. I am scared that they will take over and I will not be able to cope with my life.

My Peace: They are just feelings. I am scared of my feelings, and that is why I choose to eat instead. I don't have to address anything, explain anything, or feel anything. But I am saying they are just feelings and by acknowledging them I can accept them or let them go. I can take action such as talk with a friend if I feel that I need to. It is my choice.

To Do: To find out what you really hunger for when you are not physically hungry, do this exercise. Take a minute to turn your attention inwards. Close your eyes. Ask yourself "What am I feeling?" Perhaps you feel happy or sad, or perhaps you feel nothing. If you feel nothing, maybe it is boredom, or your

mind trying to hide your true feelings from you.
Give the feeling a name:

- ~ Excitement
- ~ Stress
- ~ Loneliness
- ~ Fear
- ~ Boredom
- ~ Sadness
- ~ Happiness
- ~ Embarrassment
- ~ Anger
- ~ Confusion
- ~ Hurt
- ~ Mischievousness
- ~ Something else?

Now ask: "What do I really want?" Is it:

- ~ Fun
- ~ Love
- ~ Company
- ~ Protection
- ~ Relaxation?

Then ask "What can I do next?" You can still eat
if you want to, but at least you have identified that

you are not physically hungry. You have a reason for feeling this way and you have identified it.

What you do next may mean doing some deeper work or seeking help from a professional. Be curious about this feeling and don't deny it for what it is. It is part of **YOU!**

Don't beat yourself up. Believe me, I have been the expert at beating myself up. Just greet the feeling, call it by its name: "Hello, Sadness, I see you are joining me again today." If it is a recurring feeling, ask yourself, "What is this about?" You have the answers within. You just have to listen.

Essential Oil Support: Roman Chamomile, Geranium, Bergamot, Rose.

Insight into Peace 12

Fear

My War: I held onto my diet and food obsession for a long time, because it was scary to consider that I would give it up forever. I asked myself "What if I couldn't cope without food obsession and diets?" I was scared that I would put on more weight and never be thin.

My Peace: I recognise my fear yet I break free anyway! I realise that fear is my personal reaction. My fear wants me to stay where I am and not move forward.

To Do: On some paper write the title "What is Stopping Me?" Allow yourself to write as much as you need to without thinking, about the blocks that are stopping you. Now imagine all these blocks being lifted, one by one. Now is the time to feel it, live it, be it and act as if you are living a life without your food and diet obsession.

Essential Oil Support: Sandalwood, Frankincense, Orange, Lavender.

Insight into Peace 13

Real Pain

My War: When I felt emotional pain I wanted to numb it out. Food became my focus. I knew I was close to an issue if I had a **sudden** urge to eat. This told me something was going on.

My Peace: Working on the issue is the only way to stop avoiding it. If we eat when we have no real physical hunger, it means that we are avoiding an issue. Even if I have given in and eaten, I can use this as a learning experience so that I can understand and recognise the issue next time it arises.

To Do: Think of a time where you ate when you had no real physical hunger. Get a large piece of paper and some crayons. A3 size paper and oil crayons are best. Ask yourself, "How do I feel about this right now?" Think of any colours, lines or shapes that go with this. Is there a symbol that comes to mind? Start drawing.

Do not be concerned with your artistic ability or lack thereof. Don't worry whether it makes sense or not. Just keep drawing until you feel that the picture is complete.

On another sheet of paper or in your journal write a list of words that go with the picture, and then answer these questions:

- ❧ How do you feel when you look at the drawing?
- ❧ Can you think of other situations when you felt like this?
- ❧ When was the FIRST time you felt like this?

Lastly, affirm that you are willing to release the issue by saying and writing "I release the past with peace and love."

If you have more feelings to release, do this by writing more in your journal, going for a walk, or meditating.

Essential Oil Support: Nutmeg, Roman Chamomile, Lavender, Melissa.

Insight into Peace 14

Grounding and Centring

My War: My thoughts consumed me. I allowed my focus to become tainted with old thoughts like "I'm too fat" or "I can't do this." I lived in my head. I did not live in the present.

My Peace: When I feel grounded and centred, food thoughts are not a priority to me. I do what I want and feel free to be myself. I am contented with life. I can say that I love myself without feeling any pain or doubt. I make sensible food choices when I have real physical hunger. My peacefulness makes my life balanced.

To Do: This exercise is best done outside with Mother Earth under your feet.

Stand barefoot, with both feet flat on the ground. Place one hand on your naval. Close your eyes and breath in to the point where you can feel your hand rising. Then as you breathe out, allow all the air to escape naturally until your hand falls. Allow your chest and shoulders to open naturally and comfortably. Feel the breath at your naval. This is your centre—your strength. Imagine each time you exhale that the energy is moving down your legs and out through the soles of your feet, grounding you to the Earth. Imagine that this energy is growing tree roots from the soles of your feet, burrowing down into the Earth to support and stabilise you. You are centred and grounded.

Practice often and the feeling will come naturally when you need it. You can call on your centring and grounding at any time when you need to get out of your head and back into your body.

Essential Oil Support: Fennel, Rosewood, Patchouli, Clary Sage.

Insight into Peace 15

Inner Child

My War: There were aspects of my childhood that caused me pain. I felt neglected by my father and smothered by my mother. I learnt patterns in childhood that I have taken into adulthood.

My Peace: I have an inner child who longs to be nurtured. I am finally acknowledging her and giving her the love she needs. The inner child must feel safe to express its full self.

To Do: Close your eyes and imagine yourself as a child. See your adult self walk over to the child and tell her she is safe. Give her a hug and promise to stay with her.

Your adult self is here to look after the child.

You are going to have some fun!

You have the choice to be as free as you want and do whatever you want.

Imagine you are flying a kite, dancing, rolling around on the grass, or building a sandcastle at the beach. Choose one of these activities and plan to act it out in real life during the coming week. Write it in your diary and make the commitment. List in detail what you will do and where you will do it. Make it a special event just for you. After your inner child experience describe your feelings in your journal. Allow yourself to nurture your inner child.

Essential Oil Support: Helichrysum, Lavender, Melissa, Roman Chamomile.

Insight into Peace 16

Eating to Cover Emotions

My War: When I ate to cover my emotions I was drawn to foods that were high in fat, salt, and sugar. I was drawn to processed food that was full of additives. I didn't care what I put into my body; I felt that I had to punish myself. I ate until I felt physically sick. The purpose of eating was to fill myself so that all I could think about was how disgusted I was with myself. I no longer had to deal with the issue at hand.

My Peace: Sometimes I eat when I am not physically hungry because of the emotions I am experiencing, but I do it thoughtfully. I make sure the food I choose is good quality food that I love. (See *Insight into Peace 2*) Then I make a *conscious decision* to eat this food as I would when I am physically hungry. This means preparing the food, placing it in a bowl or plate, sitting at the table, using cutlery, and eating with the intention of filling my body with high quality fuel.

To Do: Next time you choose to eat when you are not physically hungry, consider this: Make a *conscious decision* that you will eat the food in peace. To do this prepare your food on a special plate, set the table, sit down to eat and take one bite at a time, focussing on what is so good about this food. What need is this food satisfying right now that you couldn't satisfy from other sources?

Decide if the food is fulfilling that need. You don't have to judge yourself. Just be curious about this food and the emotions it may be connected to. The type of food you have chosen may give you a clue to the emotion. For example, if the food is crispy and crunchy, you may be trying to destress— biting down on crunchy food helps release tension. If it is sweet and gooey, you may be treating yourself because no one else will. You may be using food as a substitute for love. Examine the food and try to match it with an emotion. Write this down in your journal for further reflection at a later date. If you do this each time you will see a pattern emerge. This will help you identify the feelings which you need to examine more closely.

Essential Oil Support: Rose, Jasmine, Geranium, Benzoin.

Insight into Peace 17

Nurture Yourself

My War: I didn't like to spend time on myself. It was easier to make life busy, to focus on other people and the world beyond my emotions. When I didn't spend time on myself I nurtured myself with food. Of course, this was not real nurturing. I knew it would lead to pain. I knew I would beat myself up for overeating. I thought I deserved food as my treat to myself.

My Peace: I nurture myself with non-food pleasures. I tune in to what I need and then I make sure I put it on my agenda. It may be taking time out to read a book, to take a stroll at the beach, or to make a relaxing blend of essential oils. I understand that I deserve this time. It is not a luxury. It is a necessity for my own wellbeing.

To Do: Spend some time thinking about what *you* want. Make a list of nurturing activities. Divide them into three categories:

1. Activities that require little or no money or time.

2. Activities that require some money and extra time.
3. All day nurturing (which may need money).

Examples of activities that require little money or time are: going for a walk, reading a chapter of a book, or playing a favourite CD and doing nothing. Activities that cost some money include buying some essential oils and doing some blending, going to the markets, or having a massage. Examples of all day nurturing are going to the beach for the day, or planning a day of body pampering. You may arrange this at home, or you may visit a professional day spa. I also enjoy horse riding, so this is my ultimate all day nurturing activity.

Keep your list on hand so you can plan some nurturing activities on a regular basis.

Essential Oil Support: Lavender, Geranium, Petitgrain, Ylang Ylang.

Insight into Peace 18

The Body Knows

My War: I used look in the mirror and all I would see was fat. This gave me something tangible to blame. My body had betrayed me and I hated the way I looked. It was too painful for me to look beneath the surface. I would punish myself some more by staring into the mirror. I hated every aspect of the reflection looking back at me.

My Peace: I look in the mirror and I see a woman who has come so far. I see the beauty and courage in her eyes.

To Do: Say these sentences:

- I love myself.
- I am special.
- I am sexy.
- I have an abundant life.

For each sentence ask yourself:

- Is it true? Go with your first reaction.
- Where in your body do you feel this reaction?

～ Give it a colour.

～ Give it a texture: sharp, hard, or soft.

～ Can you name it?

Now let's examine it from a different perspective. Imagine that you have the ability to make this feeling into something new and exciting.

～ Can you change the colour to soften it and make it real?

～ Soften its texture until it feels comfortable.

～ Now is the time to choose an essential oil to match this feeling. Smell the oil and connect with your new feeling. Repeat the sentences above.

Essential Oil Support: Sandalwood, Ginger, Frankincense, Cinnamon.

Insight into Peace 19

Core Beliefs

My War: My core belief was that I was hopeless. Even when I was successful I thought I was still not good enough to meet my high expectations, or the expectations of anyone else. I felt this hopelessness at my inner core. Sometimes it screamed out at me.

My Peace: I have come to recognise that the word "hopeless", into which I put so much emotion, is just a word. It only has meaning when I give it my time and energy.

To Do: Take some time to ground and centre yourself (see *Insight into Peace 14)*. Look deep inside to identify your core belief. You may have more than one, so focus your attention on the strongest belief. Name this belief. Is it:

- Hopeless
- Useless
- Worthless
- Dumb
- Or is it something else?

Say the word over and over for a few minutes until it loses all its power. Recognise it as just a word, not as your identity.

Essential Oil Support: Juniper, Petitgrain, Rose, Roman Chamomile.

Insight into Peace 20

Resistance to Change

My War: There were days when I felt that I just didn't want to consider the idea of peace. I wanted to be able to forget my feelings and cover them up. I just focussed on food and nothing else. I didn't want to try anymore.

Even though all these thoughts caused conflict within, I didn't want to change. I wanted to stay in my food comfort zone.

My Peace: Fluctuations in my thought processes are natural. Sometimes I will feel that it is safer to go back to the food comfort zone. When I allow those feelings to surface, I can acknowledge them. This diffuses the intensity of the thought.

To Do: Take a moment to notice the feelings that arise when you visualise change.

Light a candle and focus on the flame. See how it fluctuates, how it grows weaker and then stronger. Take your thoughts fully to the candle. Meditate on the flame. Allow the flame to be your thought. Then affirm, "As the flame becomes stronger so does my willingness to change become stronger." Spend some time connecting with your feelings and the power of the affirmation. Write any thoughts or insights in your journal.

Essential Oil Support: Black Pepper, Cinnamon, Clove, Bergamot.

Insight into Peace 21

Self Loathing to Self Love

My War: I hated my food and diet obsession. I always blamed my lack of discipline around food on my inability to control myself. I thought that I had nothing to offer and that only my food and diet focus would make me feel good about myself. However, feeling good was only temporary as I would find myself in a binge, and the cycle of self-loathing would start all over again.

My Peace: I love myself for who I am and I am not ruled by my diet or food obsession. I focus on who I truly am on the inside.

To Do: Spend a day going through all your clothes, make-up, and hair products and decide which suit you and your personality. Throw out or give away any good or old clothes that don't serve you anymore. Buy new underwear and bras that fit properly. Wear clothes with pride and joy, no matter what your size. Visualise this transformation moving within you as you change the outer you.

Essential Oil Support: Rose, Ylang Ylang, Orange.

Insight into Peace 22

Body Wise

My War: My body looks like a war zone. It has many scars, bumps and lumps—a legacy of years of dieting and binging. I always hid my body in shapeless dresses and elasticised waist pants. I was ashamed of my body.

My Peace: I have my own style. I like to wear colours that suit me. My biggest achievement was buying a pair of jeans. I hadn't worn jeans for nearly twenty years. I love the casual feel of jeans. I also like white skirts! I can wear what I want, when I want.

To Do: Ask yourself what you think of your body. Is your instant reaction embarrassment or shame? Do you cover up or wear black all the time? Go online or visit a local store that has a stylist. There are websites where you can create a virtual body based on your own measurements and "dress" the model in different styles online. Find what suits you and flatters your figure type. Keep this in mind next time you buy.

Essential Oil Support: Orange, Lavender, Melissa.

Insight into Peace 23

What is Holding You Back

My War: I stayed in a violent relationship for five years and was on a binge for nearly the whole time. I did not want to move out of that comfort zone. I was overcome by "What ifs?" so food helped me to cope with my feelings. The problem was that food wasn't the answer to the situation.

My Peace: When you hit rock bottom the only way is up. The pain must outweigh the comfort zone for you to discover your way forward. My pain became too great. I know that I learnt a lot from that experience, so when I feel stuck I ask myself "What is the next thing I can do in this hour, today, or this week to move forward?"

To Do: Think of a situation where you felt that you were being held back. Take a minute to connect with the feelings. Think of a symbol that represents or matches this situation. Imagine the symbol in detail. Next, hold up your non-dominant hand. If you are right-handed, it will be your left hand, and vice versa. Imagine that your non-dominant hand is the symbol which represents your feelings. Ask your non-dominant hand to answer the following questions, as if you are asking the symbol: What are you for? Where did you come from? When did I first need you? What message do you have for me? Write the answers down as they come to you.

Essential Oil Support: Cypress, Lemon, Bergamot, Basil.

Insight into Peace 24

I Deserve It

My War: On occasions I would reach for a chocolate bar and I would hear the words in my mind "I deserve it." Food became my antidote for a stressful day, or my time to relax.

My Peace: I am able to recognise my needs and fulfil them. I don't need to stuff my emotions down with food, or focus on the next diet. If I feel tired, I rest. If I need to relax, I may use some essential oils. If I want to energise I go for a brisk walk. I listen to my needs.

To Do: Next time you reach for food as a treat, what feeling are you trying to create? What have you done to "deserve" this treat? You may find that you want to relax after a hard day at work, or to feel energised when you know that you have the afternoon to get through. Decide on a new non-food way to meet your needs.

Essential Oil Support: Jasmine, Benzoin, Rose, Geranium.

9

Life

NO MATTER WHAT WE THINK OR DO, life goes on. It is easy to ignore all the feelings trapped inside when life demands so much of us. When we are not at peace with food, life is more chaotic. While this means it is full of dramas, it can also be depressing.

When I ate, my life felt out of control. The more I tried to pull in the reins, by dieting or obsessing about food, the more out of control I felt. It was a constant cycle. Life wore me down; I dieted or binged; I blamed myself; I felt depressed. Then the cycle started all over again.

This chapter is about breaking that cycle. Taking some simple tasks such as getting organised, joining in and truly experiencing what life has to offer to open up to new possibilities outside the world of food and diets.

Use this chapter as a guide to making life, rather than your food and diet obsession, your first priority. Complete the *Insights into Peace* in order or as they appeal to you. Use your journal to continue to record your own insights. This is a perfect way to put together your plan for your life.

Insight into Peace 25

Being Grateful

My War: I was negative about everything in my life and couldn't see that there were great things happening, no matter what was going on. I watched the news on TV, and discussed the latest tragedy at length with my friends. I took in all the negative energy around me.

My Peace: I spend some time every day being grateful for the life I have, the opportunities that I will receive and all the things that are important to me, such as my family and friends.

To Do: Make a gratitude list. Start it with "I am grateful for ..." Add at least ten things to the list. As you continue throughout the day add anything else that comes to mind.

Essential Oil Support: Bergamot, Jasmine, Sandalwood, Petitgrain.

Insight into Peace 26

Less Stress

My War: I have a busy life. I haven't spoken to anyone recently who says their life isn't busy. I knew that my career had reached a dead end. I stayed in that job for twelve years—I would gain transfers and upgrade my skills, all the time knowing that I wasn't living my passion.

Eating and stress went hand-in-hand for me. When I ate, the issues that caused me stress went away temporarily. I focussed on food, as it was much easier to blame my eating habits than it was to address the core issue.

My Peace: When I am organised, I deal easily with unexpected things when they come up. I don't have to turn to eating to handle my stress. When I worked in education, I marked in my diary "unavailable" every day between midday and twelve-thirty. When I have deadlines I write in my diary when I need to start the project and a reminder at least two days before the deadline.

To Do: Get a diary. Buy one that fits into your bag. Organise EVERYTHING into appointment times.

Start by writing in everything you have planned already. Write meetings, lunch dates with friends, appointments—everything. Start with the essentials first, such as work and training times (if you or your children do sport), appointments and so forth. Then write lunch dates, phone calls, and dinner times into your diary.

For each entry, allow fifteen to thirty minutes more than you think you need. You are worth the extra time. Look at your diary each night, and visualise the next day going smoothly from start to finish.

Essential Oil Support: Lavender, Ylang Ylang, Sandalwood, Geranium.

Insight into Peace 27

Participation in Life

My War: Being overweight gave me an excuse not to participate in life. I didn't have to think about much, apart from television and food. When the kids wanted to do sport I made excuses so I didn't have to participate! I wanted their father to take them. I missed parts of their growing up. I didn't have many friends and that suited me because I didn't have to commit to social gatherings. I thought that staying at home and eating was entertainment.

My Peace: I want to be involved. I found a local women's group which I attend on a regular basis; I love the sense of connection I feel at our gatherings. I also love my work, so nothing is a chore for me. I'll happily go to an expo or run an aromatherapy class. I encourage my kids to be involved, and I take the time to be involved in their lives.

To Do: Ask yourself: "How do I participate in life?" Are there any events that you avoid, blaming it on your weight? Do you choose to opt out when given a choice to participate in a game or social event? Write the word "Participation" on a sheet of paper. Then write as many words that come to your mind as you can think of. What sorts of words come up? Are they words that describe things you want to do, or things that you want to avoid? What theme is emerging about your attitude to participation? Next, make a list of the events in which you would like to participate. You might want to start a class, or take the kids to their football game. Rate the importance of participating on a scale from one to ten. Affirm that you will follow through, and participate in these events.

Essential Oil Support: Petitgrain, Orange, Rose, Bergamot.

Insight into Peace 28

Exercise

My War: There was a time when I hadn't been for a walk for weeks or even months at a time. I felt tired and definitely didn't want to get out of bed to go for a morning walk.

My Peace: I walk most days. So what makes me do it? Before I go to bed each night, I tell myself that the next day will be awesome!

I plan ahead—I set the alarm for 6.30 a.m. so I can walk for an hour, come home, shower and prepare breakfast in time to meet my first client at 9 a.m.

Mind you, some days I don't feel so energetic. Some mornings I wake feeling tired. But because I have planned ahead, I go for my walk anyway. Walking always makes a huge difference to my day. The energy comes to me during the walk. I hear the birds sing and feel the breeze blowing against my arms. All is right with the world.

I walk in the morning because Traditional Chinese Medicine identifies 5 a.m. to 7 a.m. as the best time to exercise.

It is a time of transformation. I find it makes such a difference to my day. I used to live near the beach and going for a walk seemed to fire me up for the day ahead.

To Do: Plan a walk, a bike ride or other activity for tomorrow. If you are walking or riding, choose to take the back streets to minimise the noise and to focus on the things around you. Use the time to feel grateful:

- ∾ That you can walk or ride as far as you choose or you need to go and your legs and heart will take you.
- ∾ About the weather—the sun, the sky, the clouds, the early morning moon— whatever you can see.
- ∾ For the noises you can hear such as birds singing in the trees; or for the stillness and the silence.

So when you feel low on motivation, plan your exercise routine the night before. Organise yourself and welcome the opportunity to exercise in the morning. Know that your body will feel great and your soul will sing.

Do it for yourself, and do it because it feels good. Don't feel obliged to exercise, simply because you want to lose weight.

If walking isn't your thing, find what is. The good thing about walking is that it is doesn't cost anything (although a good pair of shoes is a bonus). You can choose where you want to walk and the time you want to spend. Focus on the parts of the body that feel good when you exercise.

Focus on your heart and the blood pumping around your body. Visualise your body being re-energised with every step. Focus on the strength that your body brings to the exercise. This will make you feel like a whole person.

Essential Oil Support: Peppermint, Bay, Coriander, Grapefruit.

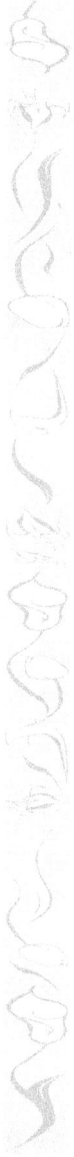

Insight into Peace 29

What Does Boredom Tell You?

My War: There are many times when I thought boredom would kill me. I was unable to allow myself some time and space. Every spare second was filled with food or diet thoughts, so I ate to fill the boredom.

My Peace: When I find I am bored I allow myself to be! These days, with the busy-ness of life I hardly have time to be bored. So any time I do feel a little jaded, I take the time to breathe and to relax. I will go and sit in the sun, or do some journaling. I allow my feelings to come out in whatever form they choose.

To Do: Next time you are bored, consider it a blessing. Use this time to relax and think about where you are in your life. You might like to write in your journal and contemplate the changes you are undertaking, or you may like to just sit in the sun!

Essential Oil Support: Coriander, Eucalyptus, Jasmine, Petitgrain.

Insight into Peace 30

Happy Place

My War: The world seemed a chaotic place to be. There was nowhere to have time for myself so I ate to relax. But I couldn't relax, because I always began to judge myself about my food obsession.

My Peace: I imagine my happy place. It gives me somewhere to go whenever I need time out. It is my place to daydream. My happy place is by the ocean. It is a beautiful white beach, with the roar of the water as the waves wash into the shore. I love the continual meditative sound of the surf. I can do whatever I please there—go for a swim, lie in the sun, or take a walk on the beach—and it all happens completely within my mind.

To Do: Find your happy place. It could be somewhere you have been before, or you can create a place that only you will ever know. Take a moment to close your eyes and think of the most beautiful place you can imagine. Is it by the ocean, in the rainforest, on top of the highest mountain or somewhere else? Imagine the feel of the sand or grass or trees. What elements of nature do you see there? Birds, a babbling spring, fish, dolphins, or something else? Imagine you are there now, in total bliss, enjoying every aspect of your happy place. Go to your happy place anytime you need some time out.

Essential Oil Support: Melissa, Jasmine, Rose, Ginger.

Insight into Peace 31

Femininity

My War: I did not know how to be feminine. I never wore makeup, and didn't spend time on myself. I didn't care about myself.

My Peace: I now do simple things that enhance my femininity. I have a skin care routine. I use pure, chemical free skin care and make up. I use essential oils as my perfume.

I express my femininity by pampering myself with natural products.

To Do: If you have never had a skincare routine, it is time to start. Make sure the products are completely natural and chemical free. Try blending some essential oil perfumes and have some fun. Make your skincare routine an expression of you.

If you currently do have a skincare regimen, check the products you are using. Do they contain sodium laurel sulphate or propylene glycol? These are chemicals.

Find a natural alternative for these products and for your perfumes. You may find that you feel better by using these natural products.

Spend some time with your products experimenting with makeup and a new skin care routine. Enjoy your natural and gorgeous femininity.

Essential Oil Support: Rose, Jasmine, Ylang Ylang, Geranium.

Insight into Peace 32

Dreams

My War: My dreams were distorted by food. I thought if I got to my goal weight by dieting that all my dreams would come true. Even when I achieved my goal weight through dieting, I wasn't happy. Worst of all, I still thought I was fat.

My Peace: I have learnt that dreams occur in the present. I am happy with who I am here and now. I know that my dreams can come true right now and my weight has nothing to do with it. I pursue all my dreams now and allow them to happen in the time they need. I don't need to monitor my weight to make my dreams come true. My dreams come true anyway.

To Do: There are two steps to allowing your dreams to happen now. The first step is to stop monitoring your weight. Get rid of the bathroom scales— donate them or pack them away. If you must weigh yourself, do it no more than once a month.

The second step is to realise your dreams now. What do you dream about? Make a list called

"Things to Do in My Lifetime." Now consider what action you need to take for each one. Prioritise the list. Give each one a completion date. The dreams can be as simple as joining a class or doing some meditation each morning.

Essential Oil Support: Helichrysum, Cedarwood, Black Pepper, Grapefruit.

Insight into Peace 33

Weigh Up Your Choice

My War: Being overweight gave me excuses. I didn't want to make the choice to eat peacefully because I didn't even think I had a choice. I felt the pressure to move on to my next diet, and worried how I would lose my excess weight. I wanted to be thin, but I could never achieve this when I was obsessing about my food and my diet.

My Peace: I made the choice to do things differently. When I finally understood that if I kept doing the same thing I would keep getting the same results, I gave up dieting forever. I know now that I can listen to my inner core. My body knows what it wants and needs. I work with my body, not against it. This choice is my peace.

To Do: Make a list of the advantages and disadvantages of continuing with your food and dieting obsession. Consider each of the items on your list to help you make your choice. Ask yourself: Is my food and diet obsession getting me what I want? Imagine eating peacefully as the alternative. How would it be different? Focus on this and write out what a typical day would look like. Act as if this day has already arrived. Keep acting until you connect with your inner core.

Essential Oil Support: Cypress, Eucalyptus, Cedarwood, Lemon.

Insight into Peace 34

Embrace the Feeling

My War: Sometimes I had just eaten and still felt so empty. I didn't know what it was. I knew that if I continued eating I would never stop, and this was my signal that something was not quite right.

My Peace: I have learnt how to embrace my hunger. When I recognise that I have emotional hunger, I use this understanding to learn more about my emotions. I understand that I need to make a choice. I can eat and continue my war with food, or I can choose to do something else and live peacefully.

To Do: Next time you have eaten and the hunger scale tells you that you are physically full, use the following sequence to determine whether you should continue eating.

1. Breathe and be still for a few minutes.
2. Ask yourself: what is my body trying to tell me?
3. Notice the area where the hunger is coming from. Is it coming from your inner core or soul?

4. Give it a colour.
5. Observe its shape and texture.
6. Ask yourself: what is my hunger about? What does it want to tell me?
7. If my hunger could speak what would it say?
8. You can choose not to eat, but instead move on to your next activity—sleep, fun, or whatever else you choose.
9. Do you still need to eat? You can choose to eat, but make it purposeful.

Essential Oil Support: Lavender, Geranium, Melissa, Benzoin.

Insight into Peace 35

Emergency

My War: Sometimes I recognised my war with food was in full swing. I knew I had no real physical hunger. I was desperate and I was searching. Food was the only thing on my mind. This is an emergency—I had to deal with my feelings, or eat.

My Peace: I need to act quickly. I need to create time and space to think. By creating time and space I can then examine what my underlying feelings were. Each time I do this I lessen the chance of another "emergency."

To Do: When you recognise the war with food has begun, STOP! You need to create some time and space between you and the kitchen. Do this by going for a walk outside, even if it is just to the garden. Move away from the food. Sit in the garden, or go for a longer walk. Take a book to read or some drawing paper or your journal.

Essential Oil Support: Lavender, Patchouli, Sandalwood, Grapefruit.

Insight into Peace 36

Connected

My War: My connection was to food. It was the one thing that I thought about constantly and it was always there for me. It felt like it was the only stable thing in my life. It was a false sense of security. It was destroying my ability to connect with anything else.

My Peace: I find my connection to my heart and my spirituality. I am connected to the universe around me. When I need to feel this connection, I go outside and spend time in nature.

To Do: Ask yourself: "How, when, where and why do I connect with food?" Write some alternative ways to get your spiritual connection such as chakra work, worshipping a deity, or grounding yourself in Mother Earth. Why is this connection important, and how does it fulfil you? Make a commitment to explore your new spiritual connection instead of connecting with food.

Essential Oil Support: Frankincense, Sandalwood, Patchouli, Cedarwood.

About the Author

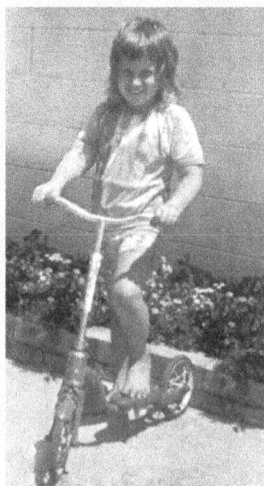

Jen was born and grew up in Brisbane, Australia. As a child she enjoyed the outdoors, especially swimming and netball. Although she enjoyed her sport, she was already starting to show signs of being overweight.

The pain of her childhood became more obvious by her size as she got older.

As a teenager, she practised extreme dieting, starving herself to thinness. Upon finishing school, she started a career in nursing. At eighteen she weighed around one hundred kilograms. Jen moved into the education sector after completing a Bachelor of Education, and became a Science and Mathematics teacher.

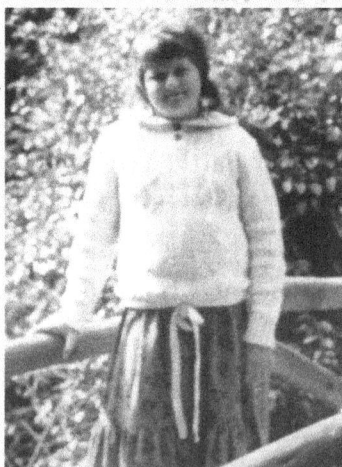

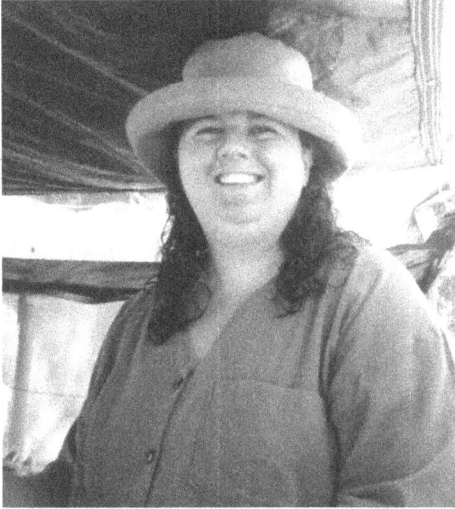

Her weight ballooned to over one hundred and twelve kilograms at twenty-eight years old.

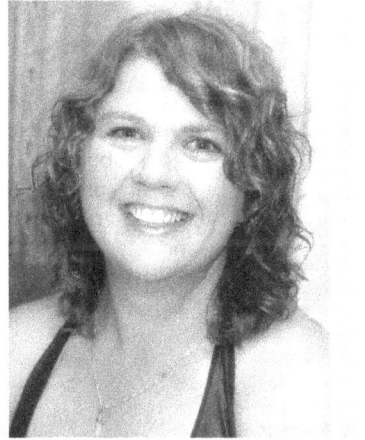

It was shortly after this Jen first started to eat peacefully. She also completed her Master's Degree in Guidance and Counselling, and worked for another four years as a school counsellor.

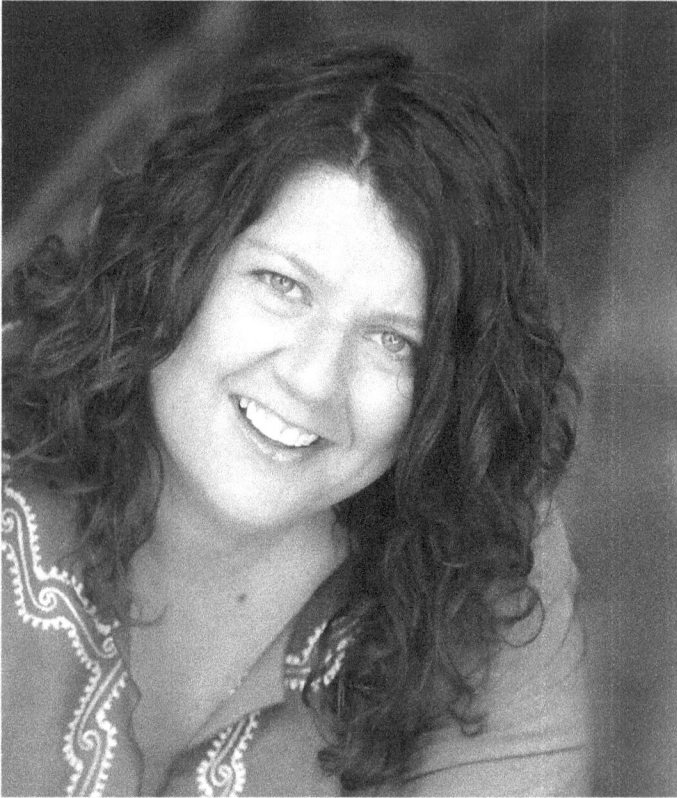

Jen has a passion for aromatherapy. She loves to educate
people about the power of essential oils, and holds
regular workshops on topics such as health, wellbeing and
aromatherapy. In the last two years she has followed her dream
and established her own business, Essential Oil Goddess. Jen
now leads a happy, confident and simple life in Brisbane with
her husband, two boys, and their dog, Bunny.

To contact Jen go to her website
www.loseweightpeacefully.com

Appendix

Essential Oil Support—How to Use Them[1]

The oils referred to in this book are all therapeutic grade essential oils. Only the purest and most helpful oils are used. Therapeutic grade essential oils are distilled at low pressure and low temperature, thereby preserving the greatest amount of chemical constituents. These are complex and active chemical constituents that are rapidly absorbed into the blood stream. This is why many clients report fast results after using therapeutic grade essential oils.

Make sure the therapeutic grade essential oils are guaranteed 100% unadulterated, chemical free, pesticide free, and organic. Please see the Resources section to find out where to purchase the highest quality essential oils. The most useful applications for essential oils are direct application, direct inhalation, diffusing and internal consumption.

Direct Application

Therapeutic grade essential oils may be applied topically in a hand or foot massage, to the points on

---

[1] PLEASE NOTE: The information presented here is not intended to replace the advice of your health care professional. Always consult with your health care professional first.

the feet, or added to bath water mixed with Epsom salts (TIP: add drops of essential oils to full cream milk, rice milk, almond milk or other milk then add to the bath for good dispersion). I use 2-3 drops in direct applications. If any oil causes redness or irritation to the skin, dilute with carrier oil such as coconut, olive or sweet almond oil.

Direct Inhalation

Put a drop of essential oil onto the palm of your hand and rub your palms together. Place your hands over your nose, close your eyes and breathe deeply. Also try inhaling through the nose, holding your breath for a count of three, and then exhaling through the mouth. Another technique is to inhale and exhale through one nostril at a time while holding the other nostril closed, and then change nostrils. If you are short of time, open the bottle, hold it up to the nose and inhale. You may also open the bottle and place it on the table or desk, allowing the vapour to penetrate the room.

Diffuse

All essential oils can be diffused on their own or in a blend. This allows the oil particles to stay suspended in the air for several hours. You should use a diffuser that does not heat the oil. Diffusers that heat the oil (e.g. with candles or electric heating) may destroy the fragile and complex chemical constituents. As a result, the oil may lose its therapeutic benefits. I diffuse approximately eight to ten drops of a single oil or a blend of oils in an ultrasonic diffuser with a timer. The diffuser automatically shuts off when a low water level is reached.

Internal Consumption

I use therapeutic grade essential oil supplements that have been approved for ingestion by the Therapeutic Goods Administration (Australia). Please check the label thoroughly and do not ingest any essential oil unless it is specified on the bottle. It is essential that you check with your qualified health practitioner before ingestion.

Resources

www.loseweightpeacefully.com

If you liked the book you will love the website.

- Download the FREE worksheet "What's Eating You?"
- Obtain bonus reader-only resources.
  Go to the **Exclusive** page at
  www.loseweightpeacefully.com and use this password:
  peace.
- Buy more copies of Lose Weight Peacefully for
  friends, family or your support group. Available
  online and delivered around the world.
- Subscribe to the FREE monthly e-zine *The Peaceful
  Way.*